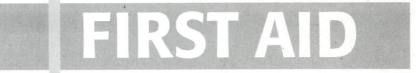

# FIRST AID

## FOR THE
# USMLE
# STEP 2 CS

# FIRST AID

# FOR THE
# USMLE
# STEP 2 CS

## TAO LE, MD

University of California, San Francisco, Class of 1996
Johns Hopkins University, Fellow in Allergy and Immunology

## VIKAS BHUSHAN, MD

University of California, San Francisco, Class of 1991
Diagnostic Radiologist

## FADI ABU SHAHIN, MD

Northwestern University
Resident in Obstetrics and Gynecology

## MAE SHEIKH-ALI, MD

Drexel University
Resident in Internal Medicine

## L. DAVID MARTIN, MD

Johns Hopkins Bayview Medical Center
Chief Resident in Internal Medicine

**McGraw-Hill**
MEDICAL PUBLISHING DIVISION

New York / Chicago / San Francisco / Lisbon / London / Madrid / Mexico City
Milan / New Delhi / San Juan / Seoul / Singapore / Sydney / Toronto

**First Aid for the USMLE Step 2 CS**

3 4 5 6 7 8 9 0 QPD/QPD 0 9 8 7 6 5

ISBN 0-07-142184-X

This book was set in Electra LH by Rainbow Graphics.
The editor was Catherine A. Johnson.
The production supervisor was Phil Galea.
Project management was provided by Rainbow Graphics.
Quebecor Dubuque was printer and binder.

This book is printed on acid-free paper.

## DEDICATION

To the contributors to this and future editions, who took time to share their experience, advice, and humor for the benefit of students.

*and*

To our families, friends, and loved ones, who endured and assisted in the task of assembling this guide.

# CONTENTS

| SECTION IV | PRACTICE CASES | 97 |
| --- | --- | --- |

# CONTRIBUTORS

**CHARLES B. ROSE, MD**
University Hospital
Former Instructor, Nuclear Medicine

**RASCHA DUGHLY, MD**
University of Maryland
Postdoctoral Program in Human Development

# Associate Contributors

**ALIREZA KHAZAEIZADEH, MD**
Associate Professor of Biochemistry
St. Luke's University School of Medicine

**BAHAR SEDARATI, MD**
Associate Professor of Pathology
St. Luke's University School of Medicine

# PREFACE

The new USMLE Step 2 CS can be a source of stress and anxiety, especially among U.S. medical students for whom this is a new requirement. *First Aid for the USMLE Step 2 CS* is our "cure" for the new exam. This book represents a virtual medicine bag of high-yield tools for students and IMGs, including:

- A thorough exam preparation guide for the new USMLE Step 2 CS. It includes proven study and exam strategies for the clinical encounters.
- Time management advice to maximize your clinical encounters.
- Step-by-step strategies for interacting with standardized patients, including "difficult patients."
- Detailed descriptions of high-yield physical exam maneuvers that will win you points without costing time.
- Minicases representing common complaints designed to help you rapidly develop a working set of differential diagnoses.
- Twenty-seven full-length cases that allow you to simulate the real exam.

This book would not have been possible without the suggestions and feedback of medical students, IMGs, and faculty members. We invite you to share your thoughts and ideas to help us improve *First Aid for the USMLE Step 2 CS*. See How to Contribute, p. xvii.

| | |
|---|---|
| *Baltimore* | Tao Le |
| *Los Angeles* | Vikas Bhushan |
| *Chicago* | Fadi Abu Shahin |
| *Philadelphia* | Mae Sheikh-Ali |
| *Baltimore* | L. David Martin |

# ACKNOWLEDGMENTS

We owe special thanks to the students and residents who helped make this project a reality: Cathleen McGill, Heather Larkin, Kurt P. Miceli, Graham Rhode Case, Joshua Leonard Shipley, Keith Thatch, Meghan Ryerson, Dora Lam, Rita Ann Kubicky, Stacey Scheib, Jean Lee, Firas Alkassab, and Sammy Mugambi. Our gratitude also goes to the attendings from Drexel University: Joseph M. Boselli, MD; Howard A. Miller, MD; Katherine Sherif, MD; David Barile, MD; and David Brody, MD.

Thanks to our editor, Catherine Johnson, for her enthusiasm, support, and commitment to the *First Aid* books. Thanks to Andi Fellows, our copy editor, for her tireless dedication to our projects, and Selina Bush for her organization and administrative assistance. For support and encouragement throughout the process, we are grateful to Thao Pham and Jonathan Kirsch.

# HOW TO CONTRIBUTE

*First Aid for the USMLE Step 2 CS* incorporates many contributions from students and faculty. We invite you to participate in this process.

Please send us:

- Study and test-taking strategies for the Step 2 CS exam
- High-yield case topics that may appear on future Step 2 CS exams
- Personal comments on review books that you have examined

For each entry incorporated into the next edition, you will receive a **$10 Amazon.com gift certificate** and a personal acknowledgment in the next edition. Significant contributions will be compensated at the discretion of the authors.

The preferred way to submit suggestions and corrections is via electronic mail, addressed to:

firstaidteam@yahoo.com

Otherwise, you can send entries, neatly written or typed or on disk (Microsoft Word), to: **First Aid for the USMLE Step 2 CS, P.O. Box 27, Woodstock, MD 21163, Attention: Contributions.** Please use the contribution and survey forms on the following pages. Each form constitutes an entry. (Attach additional pages as needed.)

Another option is to send in your entire annotated book. We will look through your additions and notes and will send you an honorarium based on the quantity and quality of any additions that we incorporate into the next edition. Books will be returned upon request. Contributions sent earlier will receive priority consideration for the next edition of *First Aid for the USMLE Step 2 CS*.

## INTERNSHIP OPPORTUNITIES

The author team of Le and Bhushan is pleased to offer part-time and full-time paid internships in medical education and publishing to motivated medical students and physicians. Internships may range from two to three months (e.g., a summer) up to a full year. Participants will have an opportunity to author, edit, and earn academic credit on a wide variety of projects, including the popular *First Aid* series. Writing/editing experience, familiarity with Microsoft Word, and Internet access are desired. For more information, e-mail a résumé or a short description of your experience along with a cover letter and writing sample to firstaidteam@yahoo.com.

## NOTE TO CONTRIBUTORS

All entries are subject to editing and reviewing. Please verify all data and spellings carefully. In the event that similar or duplicate entries are received, only the first entry received will be used. Please follow the style, punctuation, and format of this edition if possible. For additional space, use the back of this page. If you are submitting more than one entry, either photocopy this sheet before you write/type on it, or attach additional sheets.

# CONTRIBUTION FORM

## FOR HIGH-YIELD CASE TOPICS

Contributor Name: _____

School/Affiliation: _____

Address: _____

_____

Telephone: _____

E-mail: _____

Case Topic: _____

_____

Case Topic: _____

_____

Case Topic: _____

_____

Case Topic: _____

_____

Case Topic: _____

_____

Case Topic: _____

_____

Case Topic: _____

_____

Case Topic: _____

_____

**You will receive personal acknowledgment and a $10 gift certificate for each entry that is used in future editions.**

Please seal with tape only.
No staples or paper clips.

---------------------------------------- (fold here) ----------------------------------------

**FIRST AID FOR THE USMLE STEP 2 CS**
**P.O. BOX 27**
**WOODSTOCK, MD   21163**

---------------------------------------- (fold here) ----------------------------------------

# USER SURVEY

Contributor Name: _____

School/Affiliation: _____

Address: _____

_____

Telephone: _____

What student-to-student advice would you give someone preparing for the exam?

What would you change about the cases presented in Sections III and IV?

Is there an interesting experience during your test-taking that you would like to share?

How else would you improve *First Aid for the USMLE Step 2 CS?* Any comments or suggestions? What did you like most about the book?

**You will receive personal acknowledgment and a $10 gift certificate for each entry that is used in future editions.**

Please seal with tape only.
No staples or paper clips.

------------------------------------ (fold here) ------------------------------------

**FIRST AID FOR THE USMLE STEP 2 CS**
**P.O. BOX 27**
**WOODSTOCK, MD  21163**

------------------------------------ (fold here) ------------------------------------

# Guide to the USMLE Step 2 CS

▶ Introduction

▶ USMLE Step 2 CS—The Basics

▶ Preparing for the Step 2 CS

▶ Test-Day Tips

▶ First Aid for the IMG

Since 1998, all international medical graduates (IMGs) have been required to pass a clinical skills exam known as the Clinical Skills Assessment, or CSA—a test involving clinical encounters with "standardized patients"—as a prerequisite to entering residency training in the United States. With the introduction of the USMLE Step 2 Clinical Skills (CS), however, U.S. and Canadian medical students as well as IMGs are now required to demonstrate basic clinical competencies in order to enter residency training and take the Step 3 exam.

Even if you are a seasoned pro at taking standardized exams such as the USMLE Step 1 and Step 2 Clinical Knowledge (CK), you may find it challenging to prepare for the USMLE Step 2 CS—which, like the CSA it has replaced, uses live patient actors to simulate clinical encounters. Common mistakes students and IMGs make in preparing for the Step 2 CS include the following:

- Panicking because of the unfamiliar format
- Inadequate practice with mock patient scenarios prior to the actual exam
- Not developing a logical plan of attack based on patient "doorway information"
- Not understanding the required objectives for each patient encounter
- Poor time management during patient encounters
- Becoming flustered by challenging questions or situations
- Taking unfocused histories and physical exams
- Failing to understand how to interact with a patient appropriately
- Not performing easy but required patient interactions

This book will help guide you through the process of efficiently preparing for and taking the Step 2 CS with four organized sections:

- **Section I** introduces you to the USMLE Step 2 CS.
- **Section II** reviews critical, high-yield steps to take during the patient encounter.
- **Section III** provides high-yield minicases for common doorway chief complaints to help you rapidly develop focused differentials during the exam.
- **Section IV** has full-length practice cases to help you simulate the real thing.

### What Is the USMLE Step 2 CS?

The United States Medical Licensing Examination (USMLE) Step 2 CS is a one-day exam whose objective is to ensure that all U.S. and Canadian medical students seeking to obtain their medical licenses—as well as all IMGs seeking to start their residencies in the United States—have the communication, interpersonal, and clinical skills necessary to achieve these goals. To pass the test, all examinees must show that they can speak, understand, and communicate in English as well as take a history and perform a brief physical exam. Examinees are also required to exhibit competence in written English and to demonstrate critical clinical skills by writing a brief patient note (PN), some follow-up orders, and a differential diagnosis.

The Step 2 CS simulates clinical encounters that are commonly found in clinics, physicians' offices, and emergency departments. The test makes use of standardized patients, or SPs, all of whom are laypeople who have been extensively trained to simulate various clinical problems. SPs give the same responses to all candidates participating in the assessment. When you take the Step 2 CS, you will see 10 to 12 SPs, but cases will be mixed in terms of age, gender, ethnicity, organ system, and discipline. For quality assurance purposes, a video camera will record all clinical encounters, but the resulting videotapes will not be used for scoring. The cases used in the Step 2 CS represent the types of patients who would typically be encountered during core clerkships in the curricula of accredited U.S. medical schools. These clerkships are as follows:

- Internal medicine
- Surgery
- Obstetrics and gynecology
- Pediatrics
- Psychiatry
- Family medicine

It should be noted that examinees do **not** interact with children during pediatric encounters. Instead, SPs assuming the role of pediatric patients' mothers recount patients' histories, and no physical exam is required under such circumstances.

*There is no physical exam in pediatric encounters.*

## How Is the Step 2 CS Structured?

Before entering a room to interact with an SP, you will be given an opportunity to review some preliminary information. This information, which is posted on the door of each room (and hence is often referred to as "doorway information"), includes the following:

- Patient characteristics (name, age, sex)
- Chief complaint and vitals (temperature, respiratory rate, pulse, blood pressure)

You will be given 15 minutes (with a warning bell sounded after 10 minutes) to perform the clinical encounter, which will include reading the doorway information, entering the room, introducing yourself, obtaining an appropriate history, conducting a focused physical exam, formulating a differential diagnosis, and planning a diagnostic workup. You will also be expected to answer any questions the SP might ask, to discuss the diagnoses being considered, and to advise the SP about follow-up plans. After leaving the room, you will have 10 minutes to write a PN.

### How Is the Step 2 CS Scored?

Of your 10 to 12 patient encounters, 10 will be scored. Two people will score each encounter: the SP and a physician. The SP will evaluate you at the end of each encounter by filling out three checklists: one for the history, a second for the physical exam, and a third for communication skills. The physician will evaluate the PN you write after each encounter. Your score, which will be based on the clinical encounter as a whole and on your overall communication skills, will be determined in the following manner:

- **Integrated Clinical Encounter (ICE) score.** The skills you demonstrate in the clinical encounter are reflected in your ICE score. This score consists in turn of a **data-gathering (DG) score** and a **patient note (PN) score.**
  - **DG score.** To determine your DG score, SPs will document your ability to gather data pertinent to the clinical encounter. Specifically, SPs will note whether you asked the questions listed on their checklists, successfully obtained relevant information, and correctly conducted the physical exam (as indicated by the performance of the procedures on their checklists). Your final DG score will represent an average of your performance with all 10 SPs. *If you asked questions or performed procedures that are not on an SP's checklist, you will not receive credit but at the same time will not lose credit for having done so.*
  - **PN score.** A physician will score your PN according to predefined criteria, including organization, quality of information, data interpretation, legibility, and the absence of egregious or dangerous actions. Your final PN score will then represent the average of your individual PN scores over all 10 clinical encounters. Your ICE score will represent the sum of your DG and PN scores (ICE = DG + PN).
- **Communication (COM) score.** In addition to assessing your data-gathering skills, SPs will evaluate your interpersonal skills (IPS) and your proficiency in spoken English. Your IPS will be assessed on four criteria: rapport, interviewing skills, personal manner, and counseling. Your overall COM score will be the sum of your averaged IPS scores and your spoken English proficiency rating.

*ICE = DG + PN.*

The grade you receive on the USMLE Step 2 CS will be either a "pass" or a "fail." In order to pass the Step 2 CS, candidates must attain a minimum score in **both** ICE and COM. This minimum passing score, which is based on the achievement of a prespecified performance standard, is periodically reviewed and adjusted. In 2000, the passing rate for IMGs taking the old CSA was 80.4%. IMGs who were U.S. citizens fared better (87.1% passing rate) than did non-U.S.-citizen IMGs (78.7% passing rate). Pass rates have increased in 2001 and 2002 (see Table 1-1).

**Table 1-1.  CSA Pass Rates for IMGs**

|  | 2001 | 2002 |
| --- | --- | --- |
| CSA tests given | 7,240 | 8,964 |
| Pass rate for first-time takers | 84% | 82% |

In recent pilot studies, U.S. students were found to have performed at the same level as IMGs whose native language was English.

- The mean performance of U.S. students was lower than that of IMGs in the area of clinical skills.
- The mean performance of U.S. students was higher than that of IMGs in the area of communication skills.

Using the Educational Commission for Foreign Medical Graduates' (ECFMG's) pass-fail standards, the passing rate of U.S. students was slightly higher than that of first-time IMG test takers, whose passing rate was 83.3%.

*U.S. students and IMGs had similar passing rates in Step 2 CS pilot studies.*

### How Do I Register to Take the USMLE Step 2 CS?

To register for the Step 2 CS, you must have obtained a passing score on the USMLE Step 1. You should also bear in mind that registration information and procedures are constantly evolving. For the most current information on registering for the USMLE Step 2 CS, go to www.usmle.org or check with your dean's office. IMGs should also refer to the Web site of the ECFMG at www.ecfmg.org.

**For U.S. and Canadian medical students,** the registration fee for the USMLE Step 2 CS is $975 (at least through June 2005). Students will register using the National Board of Medical Examiners (NBME) Interactive Website for Applicants and Examinees (click the appropriate link at www.nbme.org). **For IMGs,** the registration fee is currently $1200. IMGs can either apply online using the ECFMG's Interactive Web Application (IWA) at http://iwa.ecfmg.org or download the paper application from the ECFMG Web site and mail it to the ECFMG along with the registration fee. Although there is no specific application deadline, you need to apply early to ensure that you get your preferred test date and center.

After your application has been processed, you will receive a scheduling permit by e-mail as well as a CD containing an orientation manual and a video of sample encounters. You will then be eligible to take the Step 2 CS for one year, starting when you are entered into the scheduling system to take the exam. Your scheduling permit will list your eligibility period, scheduling instructions, and identification requirements for admission to the exam. You can schedule the test either through the NBME or ECFMG Web sites or via telephone. Access information will be included with your registration materials. Note that test centers offer both morning and afternoon sessions. You may be offered an afternoon session if you select a date and center for which morning sessions are already filled. Try to select a date and center that will allow you to have a morning session (when you are fresher and more relaxed).

Although you cannot extend your eligibility period for the Step 2 CS, you can reschedule your exam date. The fee is $50 if rescheduling is done more than 30 days before the original test date, $150 if it is done within 30 days, and $400 if it is done after a missed test date but within the eligibility period.

### Where Can I Take the Exam?

The Step 2 CS will be administered at five regional centers (see Figure 1-1). Additional centers are currently under consideration.

For detailed information about cities, hotels, and transportation, please refer to the USMLE Web site (www.usmle.org) or the ECFMG Web site (www.ecfmg.org).

### How Long Will I Wait to Get My Scores?

Step 2 CS results are reported by "snail mail" (not by phone, fax, or e-mail) six to eight weeks after your exam date. If you do not receive your results within that time, you must send a written request for a duplicate report to the NBME or the ECFMG. As mentioned above, the score report you receive will indicate only whether you passed or failed the exam. The numerical score you achieved will not be disclosed to you or to any of the programs to which you apply. Once you pass the Step 2 CS, your passing score will remain valid for the purpose of applying for residency training.

**FIGURE 1-1. Step 2 CS Test Centers, 2004**

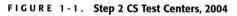

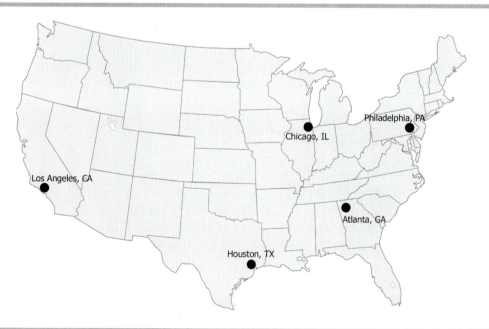

## What If I Fail?

If you fail the Step 2 CS, you can retake it. However, you must wait at least 60 days before doing so, and you cannot take the exam more than three times within any 12-month period. In addition, each time you take the Step 2 CS, you must submit a new application along with the appropriate fee. Although you are not permitted to retake the Step 2 CS during a waiting period, you can reapply for the exam during this period.

If for some reason you feel that you unfairly received a failing score, you may be able to appeal and request a rescoring of your exam. However, this is unlikely to change your overall exam results. Check your orientation manual or with the USMLE and/or ECFMG Web sites for the latest reexamination and appeal policies.

### ▶ PREPARING FOR THE STEP 2 CS

In preparing for the Step 2 CS, keep in mind that you will need to demonstrate certain fundamental but critical clinical skills in order to pass. These skills include:

- Interacting with patients in a professional way
- Taking a good medical history
- Performing an appropriate physical exam
- Counseling and delivering information
- Writing a logical and organized patient note

In this section, we will briefly explore a few of the skills delineated above. Section II will review these skills in greater detail along with the mechanics of the clinical encounter and PN.

### Ability to Interact with Patients in a Professional Way

There are several elements that you must incorporate into each encounter. These are simple and easy to learn but require practice.

- **Introducing yourself to the patient.** When you first meet a patient, be sure to smile, address the patient by his or her last name (e.g., Mr. Jones), introduce yourself clearly, shake hands firmly, and establish good eye contact.
- **"Draping manners."** Always keep the patient well draped. You can cover the patient at any time before the physical examination, but it is better to do so at the beginning of the encounter. Don't expose large parts of the patient's body at the same time; instead, uncover only the parts that need to be examined, and only one at a time. Be sure to ask permission before you uncover any part of the body, and explain why you are doing so. You should also ask permission to untie the patient's gown and should tie the gown up again when you are done.
- **Appearance.** In your encounters, you should appear confident, calm, and friendly but at the same time serious and professional. You should also

wear a clean white lab coat along with professional-looking but comfortable clothes. Do not wear shorts or jeans. Men should wear slacks, a shirt, and a tie. Women should consider slacks and low-heeled shoes and should avoid high heels and miniskirts.

- **Appropriate use of body language.** During the clinical encounter, look the patient in the eye, smile when appropriate, and show compassion. You may place your hand on the patient's shoulder or arm but not on his leg or hand when you are trying to console him. Do not exaggerate your facial expressions in an effort to convince patients that you empathize with them. Never talk to a patient while standing somewhere he can't see you, especially during the history and closure.

- **Attitude toward the patient.** Always concentrate on your patient. Ask permission before you examine any part of his body, and provide explanations of what you intend to do. Pay attention to everything the patient says and does, because it is most likely purposeful. You can show concern by:

  - **Keeping the patient comfortable.** Help the patient sit up, lie down, and get onto and off the examination table. Do not repeat painful procedures.

  - **Showing compassion for the patient's pain.** If the patient does not allow you to touch his abdomen because of severe pain, say, "I know that you are in pain, and I want to help you, but I need to examine you to be able to locate the source of pain and give you the right treatment."

  - **Showing compassion for a patient's sadness.** To demonstrate empathy, you may take a brief moment of silence and place your hand lightly on the patient's shoulder or arm. You may then say something like "I know that you feel sad. Would like to tell me about it?"

  - **Respecting the patient's beliefs.** Do not reject a patient's beliefs even if they sound incorrect to you. If a patient tells you, "I am sure that the pain I have is due to colon cancer," you may say something like "That may well be one possibility, but there are other possibilities that we need to consider as well."

### Ability to Take a Good Medical History

The interviewing techniques you use should be effective enough to allow you to collect a thorough medical history. It is true that you can prepare a list of questions to use for every system or complaint. You should be aware, however, that you will not be able to cover everything. You should thus aim to choose only those questions that are most relevant to the case at hand so as to direct the interview toward exploring the chief complaint and uncovering any hidden complaints.

If you feel that a patient is getting lost with your line of questioning, be careful, because it may indicate that you are drifting away from the correct diagnosis. You should also bear in mind that physical findings may be feigned and may not look the same as real ones (e.g., faking wheezing during chest auscultation). In such circumstances, you should pretend that the findings are real.

Do not be intimidated by angry patients. Remember that SPs are only actors, so stay calm, firm, and friendly. Ask about the reason for a patient's anger or complaint, and address it appropriately. Do not be defensive or hostile. If you do not understand what a patient has said or recognize a drug that has been prescribed, do not hesitate to ask, "Can you please repeat what you said?" or "What is the name of that drug again?"

Finally, remember to use the **summary technique** at least once during the interview. This technique, which involves briefly summarizing what the patient has just told you, may be used either after you finish taking the history or following the physical exam. Doing so will help ensure that you remember the details of the history before you leave the room to write the PN.

### Ability to Counsel and Deliver Information

At the end of each encounter, you will be expected to tell the patient about your findings, offer your medical opinion (including a concise differential diagnosis), describe the next step in diagnosis, and outline possible treatments. In doing so, you should always be clear and honest. Tell the patient only the things you know, and don't try to render a final diagnosis. Make sure the patient understands what you are saying, and avoid the use of complex medical terms. Before you leave, ask the patient if he still has any questions. After you respond, follow up by asking, "Did that answer your question?"

When counseling a patient, always be open. Tell him what you really think is wrong, and explain that the final diagnosis can be made only after some tests have been taken. You should also explain some of the tests you are planning to conduct. Address any concerns the patient may have in a realistic manner, and never offer false reassurances.

### ▶ TEST-DAY TIPS

The Step 2 CS is a one-day exam. You will be scheduled for either the morning or the afternoon session. The duration of the Step 2 CS, including orientation, testing, and breaks, is approximately eight hours. Once you have entered the secured area of the assessment center for orientation, you may not leave that area until the examination has been completed. During this time, the following conventions should be observed:

- You may not use cell phones or beepers at any time during the exam. Digital watches are allowed.
- The morning session starts at 8 A.M. and the afternoon session at 3 P.M. Test proctors will generally wait up to 30 minutes for latecomers, so the actual exam generally does not begin until 8:30 A.M. or 3:30 P.M. Nonetheless, you should plan to arrive 30 minutes before your session is scheduled to begin.
- Don't come to an afternoon session early in an attempt to meet candidates from the morning session, as they aren't allowed to leave until you are locked in.

- Bring a government-issued photo ID (e.g., a U.S. driver's license or a passport) that carries your signature.
- Be sure to bring your admission permit! You will not be admitted to the test center without it.

After the 30-minute waiting period has elapsed, the staff will give you a name tag, a numbered badge to be worn around your arm, a pen, and a clipboard. There is no need to bring a pen of your own, as you are not allowed to use anything other than the pen provided at the exam site.

Do not bring any of your luggage, as the staff will not store it for you. The staff will provide you with nothing more than a coat rack and a small storage locker for belongings that you are not allowed to carry during the encounter, such as cell phones, purses, and handbags. If you are planning to travel immediately after the exam, you can keep your luggage at the front desk of the hotel where you stayed the night before.

At the outset of your session, you will be asked to sign a confidentiality agreement. An orientation session will then be held to introduce you to all the equipment that you will find in the examination rooms. You are allowed to examine such equipment and to become familiar with it, especially the bed, foot extension, and head elevation. Do not hesitate to try every piece of equipment made available to you during the orientation session.

You will be given two breaks during the exam. The first is for 30 minutes and takes place after the fourth encounter. During this break, the staff will serve you a meal. The second break is 15 minutes long and takes place after the eighth encounter. Use the bathroom during these breaks, as you will not have time to do so during the encounters. Finally, remember that smoking is strictly prohibited not only during the exam but also during breaks. You cannot leave the center during break periods.

In the break room, you will be assigned a seat and a desk. You can keep your food or drink on this desk so that it will be accessible during break time. Although the testing staff will provide you with one meal, you may want to bring some high-energy snacks for your breaks. Also remember that your personal belongings will not be accessible to you until the end of the exam—so if you do plan to bring some food along with you, keep it on your assigned desk, not in the storage area.

The Step 2 CS is not a social event, so when you meet with other candidates during breaks, do not mention anything about the cases you just encountered. Never speak with anyone in a language other than English, as this may be considered irregular behavior.

Finally, even though all your encounters are videotaped, it bears repeating that these tapes are not used for scoring purposes. To the contrary, they are used only to ensure the safety of the SPs and candidates as well as to allow for

*Don't bring your luggage. Check it with the hotel front desk.*

quality monitoring. So don't worry about the camera, and don't try to look for it during the encounters. Instead, act as you would on a regular clinic day.

## Some Final Words

The following general principles will also help you excel on the Step 2 CS:

- **"Don't think about the past; think about the present."** Clear your head when moving to the next encounter. Thinking about what you should have done or should have asked will only distract you from your current encounter.
- **"Passing does not require perfection."** You need not be perfect. In fact, given the time constraints involved, the Step 2 CS rewards efficiency and relative completeness over perfection.
- **"There is a reason for everything you see."** If a patient is wearing a peculiar Mexican hat, inquire why this is the case. He might have been in Mexico, and the diarrhea he presents with may thus be a simple traveler's diarrhea.

### ▶ FIRST AID FOR THE IMG

If you are an IMG candidate seeking to pass the Step 2 CS, you must take a number of variables into account, from plotting a timetable to mastering logistical details to formulating a solid test preparation strategy.

## Determining Eligibility

Before contacting the ECFMG for a Step 2 CS application, you must first take several preliminary steps. Begin by ascertaining whether you are eligible to take the Step 2 CS (see Table 1-2). Check the ECFMG Web site for the latest eligibility criteria.

**TABLE 1-2. IMG Eligibility for the USMLE Step 2 CS**

| MEDICAL STUDENTS | MEDICAL SCHOOL GRADUATES |
|---|---|
| You must be enrolled in a foreign medical school listed in the International Medical Education Directory (IMED, http://imed.ecfmg.org) both at the time you apply and at the time you take the assessment. You must also be within 12 months of graduation when you take the exam. | You must be a graduate of a medical school that was listed in the IMED at the time of your graduation. |
| You must have passed the USMLE Step 1 or its equivalent before applying. | |
| You **do not** have to have passed the English language proficiency test or the Test of English as a Foreign Language (TOEFL) to be eligible for the Step 2 CS. | |

Once you have established your eligibility to take the exam, you will also need to factor in the residency matching process. If you are planning to apply for a residency in the United States, your timetable should reflect that and should be carefully planned at least one year in advance.

Bear in mind that you are allowed to **register** (pay the fee) for the Match regardless of your ECFMG status. In order for you to **participate** in the Match, however, the National Residency Matching Program (NRMP) requires that you be ECFMG certified (or that you meet ECFMG requirements for certification even if you have not received your certificate) by the rank-order-list deadline (typically in February of each year). Otherwise, applicants will be automatically withdrawn from the Match.

As a result, the ECFMG specifies a deadline by which an IMG must have taken the Step 2 CS in order to be eligible to participate in that year's Match. This deadline changes from year to year based on the NRMP rank-order-list deadline and on the time required to report Step 2 CS scores (see Figure 1-2).

**Figure 1-2. Typical Step 2 CS Timeline for IMGs**

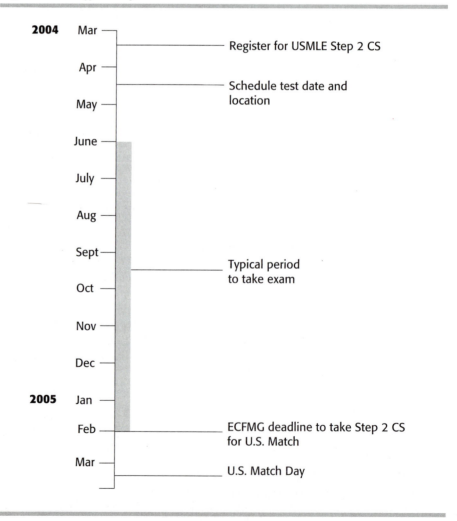

For example, January 31, 2004, was the deadline to participate in the 2004 Match.

Of course, you can still take the exam after this date if you are not planning to participate in the Match or if you are planning to sign a contract outside the Match. In order to plot your timetable, you should thus begin by checking the ECFMG's Step 2 CS deadline for the year in which you are planning to apply.

There is a significant advantage to be gained by obtaining ECFMG certification by the time you submit your application for residency in the fall. Should you do so, programs are apt to consider you a ready applicant and may favor you over other candidates who have yet to take the Step 2 CS even if such candidates have more impressive applications. In addition, if you are certified early, you may be interested in taking Step 3 and getting your results back before the rank-order-list deadline. A good score on Step 3 can provide a perfect last-minute boost to your application and may also make you eligible for the H1B visa. In sum, you would be well advised to take the Step 2 CS as soon as you are eligible to do so (see Table 1-2). At the same time, of course, you should not take the Step 2 CS until you are confident that you are fully prepared. Remember that to get ECFMG certification, you need to pass the Step 1, Step 2 CK, and Step 2 CS within a seven-year period.

*USMLE exams need to be passed in a seven-year period for ECFMG certification.*

In deciding when to apply for the Step 2 CS, when to take it, and whether you are ready for it, you should keep the following points in mind:

- Scheduling your test date can be difficult during busy seasons. You should apply at least three months before your desired examination date. Ideally, you should aim to take the Step 2 CS in June or July in order to be certified when you apply for residency.
- You should schedule your exam on the date that you expect to be fully prepared for it. For IMGs, preparation for the exam typically requires anywhere between 1 and 12 weeks, factoring in your level of English proficiency as well as your medical knowledge and skills.
- It takes up to four weeks to receive the Step 2 CS notification of registration if you choose to apply using paper applications, but it may take as few as 10 days to receive this information if you use the IWA.
- Don't be overly concerned if you are unable to meet these theoretically ideal deadlines. Most of the programs that would have invited you for an interview if you had received your Step 2 CS result will still invite you without it.

If you are an IMG living outside the United States, you must also factor in the time it may take to obtain a visa. You don't need a visa to come to the United States if you are a U.S. or Canadian citizen or a permanent resident. Citizens of countries participating in the Visa Waiver Program (such as European Union countries) may not need to obtain a visa either. You are responsible for determining whether you need a visa (usually B1 or B2) and, having done so, for obtaining that visa, regardless of how time-consuming and difficult this may be. Before you apply to take the Step 2 CS, you should therefore:

- Check with the U.S. embassy in your country to determine whether you need a visa.
- Determine how long it will take to get an appointment at the embassy.
- Find out how long it will take to get the visa and whether a clearance period is required.
- Check travel availability to the cities in which the exam centers are located.

As proof of the reason for your visit to the United States, the ECFMG will send you a letter that you can present to the U.S. consulate in your country. This letter will be sent to you only after you apply to take the Step 2 CS (i.e., after you have paid your fee) and will not guarantee that you will be granted a visa. For this reason, it would be wise not to schedule your actual exam day until you have arrived in the United States or have at least obtained your visa.

## Application Tips

Once you have received an application form to take the Step 2 CS, be sure to read the form carefully before you start filling it out. You do not want to see your application returned to you—and thus squander valuable time—simply because you forgot to answer one or more questions or because you made a careless mistake. Common errors that result in returned written applications include the following:

- Your application is not written in ink or is illegible.
- Your application is incomplete.
- You faxed your application or sent a photocopy rather than the original document.
- Your application contains a nonoriginal signature or photograph.
- Your photograph was taken more than six months before the date you submitted the application.
- The signature of the medical school official or the notary public is more than four months old.
- The medical school or notary public seal or stamp does not cover a portion of your photograph.
- You did not explain why your application was signed by a notary public but not by your medical school official.
- Full payment was not included with the application.

Commonly encountered errors specific to IMGs include the following:

- The ECFMG does not have your Step 1 score.
- You are a medical school graduate and you did not send the ECFMG a copy of your medical diploma with two full-face photographs.

- Your medical school diploma is not in English, and you did not send a translation with it.
- The medical diploma and its translation are not stapled together, and the translator's stamp does not cover both of them together.

Once you have completed your application and have double-checked it for errors, you should make an effort to send it by express mail or courier service. To check the status of your application online, you can use OASIS (http://oasis.ecfmg.org).

### Improving Your English Proficiency

For many IMGs taking the Step 2 CS, a critical concern lies in the demonstration of proficiency in spoken English. In Step 2 CS terms, this refers to the ability to speak English clearly and comprehensibly and to understand English when the SP speaks to you.

You may not have a problem with English proficiency if you are a native English speaker, studied in a U.S. or other English-speaking school, learned medicine in English in your medical school, or have spent at least a few months or years of your life in an English-speaking country. English proficiency may, however, be the main obstacle facing IMGs at the other end of the spectrum. The good news is that most IMGs who have already passed the USMLE Step 1 have the basic English knowledge required to pass the Step 2 CS. For such candidates, the key to passing the Step 2 CS lies in organizing this knowledge and practicing. Your spoken English proficiency is based on the following skills:

- **The ability to speak in a manner that is easy for the SP to follow and understand.** Choose phrases that are simpler, more direct, and easier both for you to remember and for the SP to understand. Speaking slowly will also make it easier for SPs to understand you and will minimize the effect your accent has on your English.
- **The correct use of grammar.** The key to mastering this element is to be familiar with commonly used statements, transitions, and questions and to practice them as much as possible. This will decrease the probability that you will make significant grammatical errors.
- **Good pronunciation.** Again, the key to good pronunciation lies in practicing common statements and questions, repeating them to yourself aloud, and asking someone (preferably a native English speaker) to listen to you and correct your mistakes. The more you practice, the better your chances will be of reaching an acceptable and even a superior level of clear, comprehensible English.
- **The ability to correct and clarify your English if necessary.** You may find it difficult to practice for a situation in which an SP does not understand you and asks you for the meaning of something you have just said. Here again, however, you can avoid this situation by practicing common statements, questions, and transitions; speaking as slowly and clearly as possi-

*The key to better spoken English is to practice commonly used statements, transitions, and questions.*

15

ble; and using nontechnical words instead of complicated medical terminology. If an SP still cannot understand something you have said, simply repeat the phrase or question, or restate it in simple lay terms.

You should also make an effort to remain calm throughout your clinical encounters. If you are nervous, you may find that you mumble your words, making it difficult for the SP to understand what you are saying. So just relax and concentrate.

If you get nervous and start looking at your watch and rushing, you will further increase the likelihood of making mistakes. So remain calm and take your time. Fifteen minutes may seem like a short time to do and say all the things you think are necessary, but it will be more than enough if you follow an organized plan. In general, most of the things you have to say in the exam are the same in each encounter, so by thoroughly studying common cases and medical conditions (see Sections III and IV), you can go a long way toward overcoming this obstacle.

If you are still unsure about your mastery of English and would like to see if you have achieved the level of proficiency required to pass the Step 2 CS, the ECFMG suggests that you take the Test of Spoken English (TSE). If you score higher than 35 on this exam, you have probably attained the English proficiency level necessary for the Step 2 CS. In addition, you may consider taking the TOEFL beforehand. This is not a prerequisite to the Step 2 CS or the ECFMG certification anymore. For more information about the TSE and the TOEFL, contact:

**TOEFL/TSE Services**
P.O. Box 6151
Princeton, NJ 08541-6151
(609) 771-7100
toefl@ets.org
www.toefl.org

### Getting Observerships and Clinical Rotations

Many IMGs may also lack basic familiarity with the workings of U.S. medical schools. A clinical rotation or an observership in the United States can prepare IMGs for the Step 2 CS by introducing them to the U.S. system and, in the process, instructing them in the "American way" of taking a history, performing a physical exam, and writing PNs. Clinical rotations are also good to have on your CV when you apply for residency programs. Furthermore, if you do a good job during your rotation, you can get strong letters of recommendation, which are the most important part of your application after your USMLE scores. The more time you spend in such a rotation, the better.

If you are still a **medical student,** it should not be difficult for you to find a clinical rotation. Check the Web sites of the universities in which you are interested, and send e-mails and letters to the program director and chairman of each. If you are already in the United States, call the relevant departments and make appointments to meet with those responsible for the rotations. Most of the time such personnel will send you an application by mail. For the purposes of your residency application, however, it is highly recommended that you also do a rotation in the specialty you are interested in.

*Internal medicine and emergency medicine are the best rotations for Step 2 CS preparation.*

If you are a **medical graduate,** your mission is more difficult but not impossible. You are no longer eligible for clinical rotations (clerkships), but you can still apply for observerships and externships.

The observership is perhaps the least active function you can fill in a hospital, but it can still be highly useful. Getting an observership is not an easy task because in most hospitals, there is no such formal rotation or training program. Nonetheless, here is some advice that may help you out:

- Prepare a list of hospitals in your area or any area in which you may reside. Include all types of teaching hospitals: university, community, and VA.
- Contact people (attendings, senior residents, secretaries, administrators) whom you may know. Connections are an important way to find these unofficial rotations.
- Send e-mails and/or letters to the chairman and program director of each hospital.
- Call the offices of the chairman or program director and try to set an appointment to meet them.
- Try to look for people (attendings, residents, secretaries, administrators) who are from your country and may be able to help you. Inform them that you would be willing to pay for your malpractice insurance if necessary.
- Talk to other physicians who are doing or have done observerships, and ask them where they did so and how to apply.

During your rotation, you will "officially" be an observer, which means that you cannot touch a patient or write on charts. The only things you are officially allowed to do are observe, round with your team, answer an occasional question, present some topics, and attend conferences. On rare occasions you may manage to examine some patients and write some notes. Here is some advice for making the most of your observership:

- Show a high level of enthusiasm.
- Come early and stay late (not very late, though).
- Follow up on patients your team is taking care of, and learn everything you can about them.
- Read about the cases your team is managing.
- Chat and spend time with the patients, but always let them know that you're an observer. This is the best way to practice taking histories and improving your language skills.

- Write your own PNs and orders, ask your residents to correct them, and compare them to the official notes.
- Talk to the nurses, secretaries, and support staff. This will improve your communication skills.
- If you don't get a chance to examine patients, carefully observe the residents and medical students during the physical exam.
- Do as many presentations as you can.

Here is a brief and incomplete list of hospitals that have been known to offer observerships or externships:

- D.C. General Hospital, Washington, D.C.
- Emory University, Atlanta, GA
- Harbor Hospital, Baltimore, MD
- Providence Hospital, Washington, D.C.
- VA Medical Center, Washington, D.C.
- University of Miami, Miami, FL
- Mayo Clinic, Rochester, MN (visiting physicians program)
- Mount Sinai Hospital, Miami, FL
- Hospital of St. Raphael, New Haven, CT
- Hahnemann Hospital, Philadelphia, PA
- Maricopa Medical Center, Phoenix, AZ

**Some Final Tips**

In addition to the above, there are a few final practical measures you can take to help ensure your success on the Step 2 CS exam.

- Check and recheck the ECFMG and USMLE Web sites for the latest information about the Step 2 CS. This will help you get a clear idea about regulations, requirements, registration, examination day, and all other details concerning the Step 2 CS.
- Carefully prepare for the exam using the preparation materials included in this book.
- Check other Web sites and discussion forums. They can be a good source of information.
- Review the steps of history taking (see Section II). Choose and prepare common questions and cases (see Sections III and IV).
- Review the steps of the physical examination (see Section II). Practice the physical exam as if you were in the real exam.
- Practice writing PNs (see Section IV).

# SECTION II

# The Encounter

As previously described in Section I, the Clinical Skills (CS) examination consists of 10 to 12 clinical encounters with trained "standardized patients" (SPs), with each encounter designed to replicate situations commonly seen in clinics, doctors' offices, and emergency rooms.

▶ Doorway Information

▶ Taking the History

▶ The Physical Exam

▶ Closure

▶ How to Interact with Special Patients

▶ Challenging Questions and Situations

▶ The Patient Note

Each encounter in the Step 2 CS is 15 minutes long. You will be given a warning when five minutes remain in the session. The 15-minute period allotted for each of your interviews includes meeting the patient, taking the history, performing the physical exam, discussing your findings and plans, and answering any questions the patient might have. After that, you will have 10 minutes to summarize the patient history and physical examination and to formulate your differential diagnosis and workup plan. All this may seem overwhelming, but it need not be. This chapter will guide you through the process step by step.

Fifteen minutes should be adequate for most patient encounters as long you budget your time wisely. The most common reasons for running out of time are as follows:

- Taking an overly detailed history
- Conducting an unnecessarily detailed physical exam
- Carrying out the encounter in a slow or disorganized fashion
- Allowing the patient to stray away from relevant topics
- Failure to adequately control challenging (e.g., unresponsive, angry, crying) patients

To best manage your encounter, it is recommended that you distribute your time in the following way:

- **Doorway information** (assessing preliminary information posted on the door of each room): 10 to 20 seconds
- **History:** 7 to 8 minutes
- **Physical exam:** 3 to 5 minutes
- **Closure:** 2 to 3 minutes

*Any time saved from the patient encounter can be used to write the patient note.*

Of course, this is only an approximation of how you should divide your time during your 15-minute encounter. In reality, each encounter is different, so some will require more time for taking the history or physical while others will demand that more time be spent on closure and patient counseling. You should thus tailor your time to fit each case. Here are some additional time management tips:

- Do not waste valuable time looking at your watch or the clock on the wall. We recommend using the official announcement that five minutes remain in the encounter as your only time indicator. If you have not begun to perform the physical exam by that point, you should do so.
- An organized and well-planned history is key. Stay focused on asking questions that are pertinent to the chief complaint.
- A brief and focused physical exam is also critical. There is no need to conduct a comprehensive physical examination during encounters.
- Never try to save time by ignoring the patient's questions, requests, or emotional status.
- Practice is the best way to improve your performance, efficiency, and sense of timing.

Figure 2-1 further describes the key components and desired outcomes of the clinical encounter. The sections that follow will guide you through each of these components.

As has previously been described, you will be given a chance to review some preliminary patient information, known as "doorway information," at the outset of each encounter. This information, which is posted on the door of the examination room, includes the patient's name, age, and gender; the reason for the visit; the patient's vital signs (pulse, blood pressure, temperature in

**Figure 2-1.** **Overview of the Clinical Encounter**

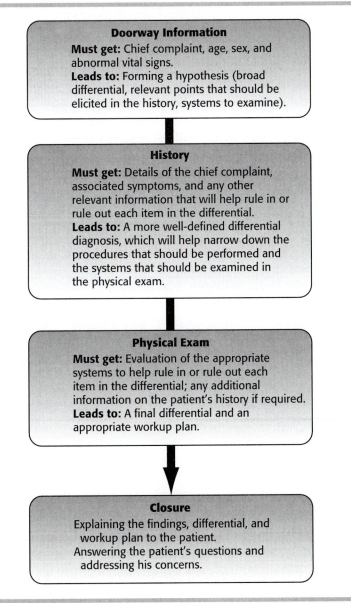

**Doorway Information**
**Must get:** Chief complaint, age, sex, and abnormal vital signs.
**Leads to:** Forming a hypothesis (broad differential, relevant points that should be elicited in the history, systems to examine).

**History**
**Must get:** Details of the chief complaint, associated symptoms, and any other relevant information that will help rule in or rule out each item in the differential.
**Leads to:** A more well-defined differential diagnosis, which will help narrow down the procedures that should be performed and the systems that should be examined in the physical exam.

**Physical Exam**
**Must get:** Evaluation of the appropriate systems to help rule in or rule out each item in the differential; any additional information on the patient's history if required.
**Leads to:** A final differential and an appropriate workup plan.

**Closure**
Explaining the findings, differential, and workup plan to the patient.
Answering the patient's questions and addressing his concerns.

both centigrade and Fahrenheit, and respiratory rate); and the task you will be called on to perform.

You should begin by reading the doorway information carefully, checking the chief complaint, and trying to organize in your mind the questions you will need to ask and the systems you will have to examine. Toward this goal, you should look for abnormalities in vital signs without trying to memorize actual numbers. Assume that these vital signs are accurate.

At this time, you should remain calm and confident by reminding yourself that what you are about to encounter is a common medical case. You should also bear in mind that SPs are easier to deal with than real patients in that they are more predictable and already know what you are expected to do. Remember that a second copy of the doorway information sheet will be available on the other side of the door, so you can review that information at the end of each encounter. Note, however, that the time you spend reading the doorway information is included in the 15-minute time limitation.

*Address the patient by his or her name when you enter the room.*

Your entrance into the examination room is also a critical part of the encounter as a whole. So before you enter the room, be sure to read and commit to memory the patient's last name. Then knock on the door and, once you have entered the examination room, say the patient's name aloud. You will receive credit for having done so and will not have to worry about remembering the patient's name for the remainder of the encounter.

After your initial entrance, you should shake hands with the patient and introduce yourself in a confident yet friendly manner (e.g., "Hi, I am Dr. Morton. Nice to meet you."). You may also add something like "I would like to ask you some questions and do a physical exam." You should make an effort to establish eye contact with the patient during this initial period.

▶ **TAKING THE HISTORY**

Your ability to take a detailed yet focused history is essential to the formulation of a differential diagnosis and workup plan. The discussion that follows will help guide you through this process in a manner that will maximize your chances of success.

### Guidelines

You may take the history while either standing in front of the patient or sitting on the stool that is usually located near the bed. You will find a sheet placed on this stool. Begin by removing the sheet and draping the patient. Doing so prior to taking the history is a good idea to guarantee your credit for that early. Don't cross your arms in front of your chest when talking to the patient, especially with the clipboard in your hands. It's best to sit down on the stool, relax, and keep the clipboard on your lap. If you decide to stand, maintain a distance of approximately two feet between yourself and the patient.

As previously described, the interview as a whole should take no more than seven to eight minutes. You can start your interview by asking the patient an open-ended question such as "So what brought you to the hospital/clinic today?" or "How can I help you today?" See Figure 2-2 to get an overview of the process.

### Additional Tips

Once the interview has begun, be sure to maintain a professional yet friendly demeanor. You should speak clearly and slowly, and your questions should be short, well phrased, and simple. Toward that end, avoid the use of medical terms; instead, use simple words that a layperson can understand. For example, don't use the term "renal calculus"; use "kidney stone" instead. If you find yourself obliged to use a medical term that the patient may not under-

**Figure 2-2.** **History-Taking Overview**

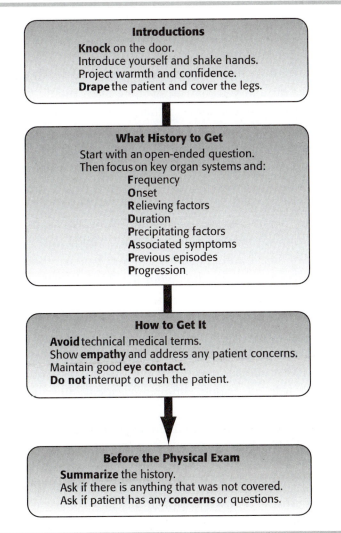

**Introductions**
**Knock** on the door.
Introduce yourself and shake hands.
Project warmth and confidence.
**Drape** the patient and cover the legs.

**What History to Get**
Start with an open-ended question.
Then focus on key organ systems and:
    **F**requency
    **O**nset
    **R**elieving factors
    **D**uration
    **P**recipitating factors
    **A**ssociated symptoms
    **P**revious episodes
    **P**rogression

**How to Get It**
**Avoid** technical medical terms.
Show **empathy** and address any patient concerns.
Maintain good **eye contact.**
**Do not** interrupt or rush the patient.

**Before the Physical Exam**
**Summarize** the history.
Ask if there is anything that was not covered.
Ask if patient has any **concerns** or questions.

*Use simple, nontechnical terminology when speaking to the patient.*

stand, try to offer a quick explanation. Don't wait for the patient to ask you for the meaning of a term, or you may lose credit.

If you don't understand something the patient has said, you may ask him either to explain his statement or to repeat it: "Can you please explain what you mean by that?" or "Can you please repeat what you have just said?" At the same time, do not rush the patient. Instead, give him the time he needs to respond. In interacting with the patient, you should always remember to ask questions in a neutral and nonjudgmental way.

You should also remember not to interrupt the patient unless it is absolutely necessary. If the patient starts telling lengthy stories that are irrelevant to the chief complaint, you can interrupt him politely but firmly by saying something like "Excuse me, Mr. Johnson. I understand how important those issues are for you, but I'd like to ask you some additional questions about your current problem." You can also redirect the conversation by summarizing what the patient has told you thus far and then moving to the next step. For example, you can say, "So as I understand it, your abdominal pains are infrequent, last a short time, and are always in the middle of your belly. Now tell me about . . ."

*Summarizing key facts for the patient will earn you credit.*

It is also critical to summarize what the patient has told you, not only to verify that you have understood him but also to ensure that you receive credit. You need to use this summary technique no more than once during the encounter in order to get credit, but you may use it more often should you consider it necessary. It is recommended, however, that you give a summary (1) after you have finished taking the history and before you start examining the patient, or (2) just after you have finished examining the patient and before you give him your medical opinion. In either case, your summary should include only the points relevant to the patient's chief complaint.

Minor transitions may also be used during the history. For example, when you want to move from the history of present illness (HPI) to the patient's past medical history or social and sexual history, you can say something like "I need to ask you some questions about your health in the past," or "I'd like to ask you a few questions about your lifestyle and personal habits."

*Look for nonverbal clues.*

To ensure that you stay on track in gathering information, you will also need to watch the patient carefully, paying attention to his every word, move, or sign. Remember that clinical encounters are staged, so it is uncommon for something to occur for no reason. Although accidents do happen (for example, a patient once started to hiccup inadvertently), most likely a patient will cough in an encounter because he is intending to convey that he has bronchitis, not because he "feels like" doing so.

By the same logic, you should address every sign you see in the patient (e.g., "You look sad; do you know the reason?" or "You look concerned; is there anything that is making you worry?"). If your patient is coughing, ask him about his cough even if he didn't mention it as the reason for his visit. If he is using a tissue, ask to see it in order to check the color of the sputum. A spot of blood on the tissue may take you by surprise!

Finally, take brief notes throughout the interview, mainly to record relevant yet easy-to-forget pieces of information such as the duration of the chief complaint or the number of years the patient smoked. The extent of your note taking inside the encounter will depend on how much you trust your memory.

Before you finish your interview and move to the physical examination, you may ask the patient something like "Is there anything else you would like to tell me about?" or "Is there anything else you forgot to tell me about?"

### Common Questions to Ask the Patient

In this section, we will cover a wide spectrum of questions that you may need to pose in the course of each of your patient interviews. This is not meant to be a complete list. You do not have to use all of the questions stated below. Instead, be selective in choosing the questions you need to obtain a concise, relevant history.

#### Opening of the encounter
- "Mr. Jones, hello; I am Dr. Singh. It's nice to meet you. I'd like to ask you some questions and examine you today."
- "How can I help you today?"
- "What brought you to the hospital/clinic today?"
- "What made you come in today?"

#### Pain
- "Do you have pain?"
- "When did it start?"
- "How long have you had this pain?"
- "How long does it last?"
- "How often does it come on?"
- "Where do you feel the pain?"
- "Can you show me exactly where it is?"
- "Does the pain travel anywhere?"
- "What is the pain like?"
- "Can you describe it for me?"
- "Is it sharp, dull, burning, pulsating, cramping, or pressure-like?"
- "Is it constant, or does it come and go?"
- "On a scale of 1 to 10, with 10 being the worst, how would you rate your pain?"
- "What brings the pain on?"
- "Do you know what causes the pain to start?"
- "Does anything make the pain better?"
- "Does anything make it worse?"
- "Have you had similar pain before?"

### Nausea

- "Do you feel nauseated?"
- "Do you feel sick to your stomach?"

### Vomiting

- "Did you vomit?"
- "Did you throw up?"
- "What color was the vomit?"
- "Did you see any blood in it?"

### Cough

- "Do you have a cough?"
- "When did it start?"
- "How often do you cough?"
- "Do you bring up any phlegm with your cough, or is it dry?"
- "Does anything come up when you cough?"
- "What color is it?"
- "Is there any blood in it?"
- "Can you estimate the amount of the phlegm? Teaspoon? Tablespoon? Cupful?"
- "Does anything make it better?"
- "Does anything make it worse?"

### Headache

- "Do you get headaches?"
- "Tell me about your headaches."
- "Tell me what happens before/during/after your headaches."
- "When do your headaches start?"
- "How often do you get them?"
- "When your headache starts, how long does it last?"
- "Can you show me exactly where you feel the headache?"
- "What causes the headache to start?"
- "Do you have headaches at certain times of the day?"
- "Do your headaches wake you up at night?"
- "What makes the headache worse?"
- "What makes it better?"
- "Can you describe the headache for me, please? Is it sharp, dull, pulsating, pounding, or pressure-like?"
- "Do you notice any change in your vision before/during/after the headaches?"
- "Do you notice any numbness or weakness before/during/after the headaches?"
- "Do you feel nauseated? Do you vomit?"
- "Do you notice any fever or stiff neck with your headaches?"

### Fever

- "Do you have a fever?"
- "Do you have chills?"
- "Do you have night sweats?"

- "Do you sweat during the night?"
- "How high is your fever?"

### Shortness of breath
- "Do you get short of breath?"
- "Do you get short of breath when you're climbing stairs?"
- "How many steps can you climb before you get short of breath?"
- "When did it start?"
- "When do you feel short of breath?"
- "What makes it worse?"
- "What makes it better?"
- "Do you wake up at night short of breath?"
- "Do you have to prop yourself up on pillows in order to sleep at night? How many?"
- "Have you been wheezing?"
- "How far do you walk on level ground before you have shortness of breath?"
- "Have you noticed any fluid retention around your ankles?"

### Urinary symptoms
- "Has there been any change in your urinary habits?"
- "Do you have any pain or burning during urination?"
- "Have you noticed any change in the color of your urine?"
- "How often do you have to urinate?"
- "Do you have to wake up at night to urinate?"
- "Do you have any difficulty urinating?"
- "Do you feel that you haven't completely emptied your bladder after urination?"
- "Do you need to strain/push during urination?"
- "Have you noticed any weakness in your stream? Any dribbling of urine?"
- "Have you noticed any blood in your urine?"

### Bowel symptoms
- "Has there been any change in your bowel movements?"
- "Do you have diarrhea?"
- "Are you constipated?"
- "How long have you had diarrhea/constipation?"
- "How many bowel movements do you have per day/week?"
- "What does your stool look like?"
- "What color is your stool?"
- "Is there any mucus or blood in it?"
- "Do you feel any pain when you have a bowel movement?"
- "Did you travel recently?"

### Weight
- "Have you noticed any change in your weight?"
- "How many pounds did you gain/lose?"
- "Over what period of time did it happen?"
- "Was the weight gain/loss intentional?"

### Appetite

- "How is your appetite?"
- "Has there been any change in your appetite?"

### Diet

- "Has there been any change in your eating habits?"
- "What do you usually eat?"
- "Did you eat anything unusual lately?"
- "What did you eat before the symptoms started?"
- "Is there any kind of special diet that you are following?"

### Sleep

- "Do you have any problems falling asleep?"
- "Do you have any problems staying asleep?"
- "Do you have any problems waking up?"
- "Do you feel refreshed when you wake up?"
- "Do you snore?"
- "Do you feel sleepy during the day?"
- "How many hours do you sleep?"
- "Do you take any pills to help you go to sleep?"

### Dizziness

- "Do you ever feel dizzy?"
- "Tell me exactly what you mean by dizziness."
- "Did you feel the room spinning around you, or did you feel lightheaded as if you were going to pass out?"
- "Did you black out?"
- "Did you lose consciousness?"
- "Did you notice any change in your hearing?"
- "Do your ears ring?"
- "Do you feel nauseated? Do you vomit?"
- "What causes this dizziness to happen?"
- "What makes you feel better?"

### Joint pain

- "Do you have any painful joints in your body?"
- "Do you have pain in any of your joints?"
- "Have you noticed any rash with your joint pain?"

### Travel history

- "Have you traveled recently?"

### Past medical history

- "Have you had this problem or anything similar before?"
- "Have you had any other major illnesses before?"
- "Do you have any other medical problems?"
- "Have you been hospitalized before?"
- "Have you had any surgeries before?"

- "Have you had any accidents or injuries before?"
- "Are you taking any medications?"
- "Are you taking any over-the-counter drugs, vitamins, or herbs?"
- "Do you have any allergies?"

### Family history
- "Does anyone in your family have the same problem or anything similar?"
- "Are your parents alive?"
- "Are they in good health?"
- "What did you mother/father die of?"
- "Are your brothers or sisters alive?"
- "Are they in good health?"

### Social history
- "Do you smoke?"
- "How many packs a day?"
- "How long have you smoked?"
- "Do you drink alcohol?"
- "What do you drink?"
- "How much do you drink per week?"
- "Do you use any illegal drugs?"
- "Which ones do you use?"
- "How often do you use them?"
- "Do you smoke or inject them?"
- "What type of work do you do?"
- "Where do you live? With whom?"
- "Tell me about your life at home."
- "Are you married?"
- "Do you have children?"
- "Do you have a lot of stressful situations on your job?"
- "Are you exposed to environmental hazards on your job?"

### Alcohol history
- "How much alcohol do you drink?"
- "Tell me about your use of alcohol."
- "Have you ever had a drinking problem?"
- "When was your last drink?"
- Administer the CAGE questionnaire:
  - "Have you ever felt a need to **cut** down on drinking?"
  - "Have you ever felt **annoyed** by criticism of your drinking?"
  - "Have you ever had **guilty** feelings about drinking?"
  - "Have you ever had a drink first thing in the morning ('**eye opener**') to steady your nerves or get rid of a hangover?"

### Sexual history
- "I would like to ask you some questions about your sexual health and practice."
- "Are you sexually active?"
- "Do you use condoms? Always? Other contraceptives?"

- "Are you sexually active? With men, women, or both?"
- "How many sexual partners have you had in the last year?"
- "Do you currently have one partner or more than one?"
- "Have you ever had an STD?"
- "Do you have any problems with sexual function?"
- "Do you have any problems with erections?"
- "Do you use any contraception?"
- "Have you ever been tested for HIV?"

### Gynecologic/obstetric history

- "At what age did you have your first menstrual period?"
- "How often do you get your menstrual period?"
- "How long does it last?"
- "When was your last menstrual period?"
- "Have you noticed any change in your periods?"
- "Do you have cramps?"
- "How many pads or tampons do you use per day?"
- "Have you noticed any spotting between periods?"
- "Have you ever been pregnant?"
- "How many times?"
- "How many children do you have?"
- "Have you ever had a miscarriage or an abortion?"
- "In what trimester?"
- "Do you have pain during intercourse?"
- "Do you have any vaginal discharge?"
- "Do you have any problems controlling your bladder?"
- "Have you had a Pap smear before?"

### Pediatric history

- "Was your pregnancy full term (40 weeks or nine months)?"
- "Did you have routine checkups during your pregnancy? How often?"
- "Did you have any complications during your pregnancy/during your delivery/after delivery?"
- "Was an ultrasound performed during your pregnancy?"
- "Did you smoke, drink, or use drugs during your pregnancy?"
- "Was it a vaginal delivery or a C-section?"
- "Did your child have any medical problems after birth?"
- "When did your child have his first bowel movement?"

### Growth and development

- "When did your child first smile?"
- "When did your child first sit up?"
- "When did your child start crawling?"
- "When did your child start talking?"
- "When did your child start walking?"
- "When did your child learn to dress himself?"
- "When did your child learn to tie his shoes?"

- "When did your child start using short sentences?"
- "When did your child start putting things in his mouth?"

### Feeding history
- "Did you breast-feed your child?"
- "When did your child start eating solid food?"
- "How is your child's appetite?"
- "Does your child have any allergies?"
- "Is your child's formula fortified with iron?"
- "Are you giving your child pediatric multivitamins?"

### Routine care
- "Are your child's immunizations up to date?"
- "When was the date of your child's last routine checkup?"
- "Has your child had any serious illnesses?"
- "Is your child taking any medications?"
- "Has your child ever been hospitalized?"

### Psychiatric history
- "Tell me about yourself and your future goals."
- "How long have you been feeling unhappy/sad/anxious/confused?"
- "Do you have any idea what might be causing this?"
- "Would you like to share with me what made you feel this way?"
- "Do you have any friends or family members you can talk to?"
- "Has your appetite changed lately?"
- "Has your weight changed recently?"
- "Tell me how you spend your time/day."
- "Do you have any problems falling asleep/staying asleep/waking up?"
- "Has there been any change in your sleeping habits lately?"
- "What interests/hobbies do you have? Do you enjoy them?"
- "Do you take interest or pleasure in your daily activities?"
- "Do you have any memory problems?"
- "Do you have difficulty concentrating?"
- "Do you have hope for the future?"
- "Have you ever thought about hurting yourself or ending your life?"
- "Do you think of killing yourself/putting an end to your own life?"
- "Do you have a plan to end your life?"
- "Would you mind telling me about it?"
- "Do you feel that you want to hurt other people? Have you ever done so?"
- "Do you ever see or hear things that others can't see or hear?"
- "Do you hold beliefs about yourself or the world that other people would find odd?"
- "Do you feel as if other people are trying to harm or control you?"
- "Has anyone in your family ever experienced depression?"
- "Has anyone in your family ever been diagnosed with a mental illness?"
- "Would you like to meet with a counselor to help you with your problem?"
- "Would you like to join a support group?"

- "What do you think makes you feel this way?"
- "Can you tell me more about it?"
- "Have you lost any interest in your social activities and relationships?"
- "Do you feel hopeless?"
- "Do you feel guilty about anything?"
- "How is your energy level?"
- "Can you still perform your daily functions or activities?"
- "Do you have any thoughts of harming yourself?"
- "Do you have any thoughts of harming others?"
- "Whom do you live with?"
- "How do they react to your behavior?"
- "Do you have any problems in your job?"
- "How is your performance on your job?"
- "Have you had any recent emotional or financial problems?"
- "Have you had any recent traumatic event in your family?"
- "Does anyone support you?"

### Daily activities (for dementia patients)

- "Tell me about your day yesterday."
- "Do you need any help bathing?"
- "Do you need any help getting dressed?"
- "What do you need help with when you are getting dressed?"
- "Do you need any help going to the toilet?"
- "Do you need any help transferring from your bed to the chair?"
- "Do you ever have accidents with your urine or bowel movements?"
- "Do you ever not make it to the toilet on time?"
- "Do you need any help feeding yourself?"
- "What do you need help with when you eat?"
- "Do you need any help taking your medications/using the telephone/shopping/preparing food/cleaning your house/doing laundry/getting from place to place/managing money?"

### Abuse

- "Are you safe at home?"
- "Is there any threat to your personal safety at home or anywhere else?"
- "Does anyone (your husband/wife/parents/boyfriend) treat you in a way that hurts you or threatens to hurt you?"
- "Can you tell me about the bruises on your arm?"

### ▶ THE PHYSICAL EXAM

### Guidelines

In this section, we will suggest a systematic way to perform the physical examination. You can use this method or any other system with which you feel comfortable. Regardless of the method you choose, however, it is essential that you practice until you can perform the physical exam without mistakes or hesitation.

As described earlier, the physical examination can take up to five minutes. Given that the history portion of the encounter is estimated to take seven to eight minutes, you should already have started the physical examination by the time you hear the announcement that you have five minutes remaining in the encounter. Bear in mind that there is no time for a complete physical exam. Instead, you should aim at conducting a focused examination to look for physical findings that can support the differential diagnosis you made after taking the history. See Figure 2-3 to get an overview of the process.

*The key is a focused physical examination.*

Before you begin, you should announce to the patient the need for the physical exam. Then, don't forget to wash your hands with soap and water and to dry them carefully. (You can wear gloves instead if you so choose.) While you are washing your hands, use the time to think about what you should examine and whether there is anything you neglected to ask the patient. You should then drape the patient if you have not yet done so. The drape will be on the stool; unfold it and cover the patient from the waist down.

Before you touch the patient, make sure your hands are warm (rub your hands together if they are cold). In a similar manner, rub the diaphragm of your stethoscope to warm it up before you use it. Do not auscultate or palpate through the patient's gown.

As you proceed, be sure to ask the patient's permission before you uncover any part of his body (e.g., "Is it okay if I untie your gown in order to examine your chest?" or "Can I move down the sheet to examine your belly?"). You may also ask the patient to uncover himself. You should expose only the area

**Figure 2-3. Physical Exam Overview**

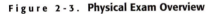

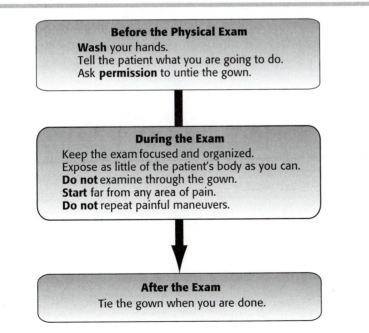

*Ask permission before touching or uncovering the patient.*

*Be alert to special situations that may occur during a patient encounter.*

you need to examine. Do not expose large areas of the patient's body at once. After you have examined a given area, cover it immediately.

During the physical exam, you will be scored both for performing a given procedure and for doing so correctly. You will not get credit for conducting an extra maneuver or for examining a nonrequired system, but failure to perform a required procedure will cost you a check mark on your list. You should also bear in mind that you are not allowed to perform a corneal reflex, breast, rectal, pelvic, or genital examination. If you think any of the above-mentioned exams is indicated, you should tell the patient that you will need to do the specific exam later and then remember to add the exam to your orders on your patient note (PN). When you have concluded a given procedure, remember to say "thank you." Then explain the next step, and ask the patient for his permission to proceed. The patient should always be made to feel that he is in control of his body.

During the physical exam, you may ask the patient any additional questions that you feel may be pertinent to the history. It is recommended, however, that you stop the physical exam while doing so in order to reestablish eye contact. After the patient has answered your questions, you may resume the exam.

Finally, you should remain alert to special situations that may not unfold as would an ordinary physical exam. When you enter the exam room, for example, the patient may hand you an insurance form requesting that only certain systems be examined. In such cases, the patient will usually tell you that you do not need to take a history. Should this occur, simply introduce yourself, proceed to examine the systems listed, and then leave the room. No PN is required under such circumstances; instead, you are required only to fill out the form the patient gave you with the appropriate findings. In such encounters, the emphasis will be on the correct performance of the physical exam maneuvers and on professional and appropriate interaction with the patient.

**Physical Exam Review**

The following is a review of the steps involved in the examination of each of the body's main systems. Included are samples of statements that can be used during the physical exam. Remember that it is crucial to keep the patient informed of what is going on as well as to ask his consent before each step.

1. HEENT exam
   - **What to say to the patient before and during the exam:**
     - "I need to examine your sinuses, so I am going to press on your forehead and cheeks. Please tell me if you feel pain anywhere."
     - "I would like to examine your eyes now."
     - "I am going to shine this light in your eyes. Can you please look at the clock on the wall?"

- ▪ "I need to examine your ears now."
- ▪ "Can you please open your mouth? I need to check the inside of your mouth and your throat."
- ▪ **What to perform during the HEENT exam:**
  - ▪ Head:
    1. Inspect the head for signs of trauma and scars.
    2. Palpate the head for tenderness or abnormalities.
  - ▪ Eyes:
    1. Inspect the sclerae and conjunctivae for color and irritation.
    2. Check the pupils for symmetry and reactivity to light.
    3. Check the extraocular movements of the eyes.
    4. Check visual acuity with the Snellen eye chart.
    5. Perform a funduscopic exam. Remember the rule "right-right-right" (ophthalmoscope in examiner's right hand—patient's right eye—examiner's right eye) and the rule "left-left-left" (ophthalmoscope in examiner's left hand—patient's left eye—examiner's left eye).
  - ▪ Ears:
    1. Conduct an external ear inspection for discharge, skin changes, or masses.
    2. Palpate the external ear for pain (otitis externa); do the same for the mastoid.
    3. Examine the ear canal and the tympanic membrane using an otoscope. (Don't forget to use a new speculum for the patient.)
    4. Conduct the Rinne and Weber tests.
  - ▪ Nose:
    1. Inspect the nose.
    2. Palpate the nose and sinuses.
    3. Inspect the nasal turbinates and the nasal septum with a light source.
  - ▪ Mouth and throat:
    1. Inspect with a light.
    2. Tooth tapping may be performed if needed.
2. Cardiovascular exam
   - ▪ **What to say to the patient before and during the exam:**
     - ▪ "I need to listen to your heart."
     - ▪ "Can you hold your breath, please?"
     - ▪ "Can you sit, please?"
     - ▪ "Can you turn to your left side, please?"
     - ▪ "I am going to examine your legs to check for fluid retention. Is that okay with you?"
     - ▪ "I need to check the pulse in your arms and legs now."
   - ▪ **What to perform during the cardiovascular exam:**
     - ▪ When examining the heart, do not lift up the patient's gown. Rather, pull the gown down the shoulder, exposing only the area to be examined.
     - ▪ Listen to the carotids for bruits (use the bell of the stethoscope).

- Look for JVD.
- Palpate the chest for the PMI, retrosternal heave, and thrills.
- Listen to at least two of the four cardiac areas. (Listen to the mitral area with the patient on his left side.)
- Listen to the base of the heart with the patient leaning forward.
- Check for pedal edema.
- Check the peripheral pulses.

3. Pulmonary exam
   - **What to say to the patient before and during the exam:**
     - "I need to listen to your lungs now."
     - "Can you take a deep breath for me, please?"
     - "Can you say '99' for me, please?"
     - "I am going to tap on your back to check your lungs. Is that okay with you?"
   - **What to perform during the pulmonary exam:**
     - Examine both the front and the back of the chest.
     - Don't percuss or auscultate through the patient's gown.
     - Don't percuss or auscultate over the scapula.
     - Allow a full inspiration and expiration in each area of the chest.
     - Inspect: The shape of the chest, respiratory pattern, deformities.
     - Palpate: Tenderness, tactile fremitus.
     - Percuss.
     - Auscultate, egophony.

4. Abdominal exam
   - **What to say to the patient before and during the exam:**
     - "I need to examine your belly/stomach now."
     - "I am going to listen to your belly now."
     - "I am going to press on your belly. Tell me if you feel any pain or discomfort."
     - "Now I need to tap on your belly."
     - "Do you feel any pain when I press in or when I let go? Which hurts more?"
   - **What to perform during the abdominal exam:**
     - Inspect.
     - Auscultate (always auscultate before you palpate the abdomen).
     - Percuss.
     - Palpate: Start from the point that is farthest from the pain; be gentle on the painful area, and don't try to reelicit the pain. Check for rebound tenderness, CVA tenderness, obturator sign, psoas sign, and Murphy's sign.
     - Check the liver span.

5. Neurologic exam
   - **What to say to the patient before and during the exam—mini-mental status exam questions:**
     - "I would like to ask you some questions to test your orientation."
     - "I would like to check your memory and concentration by asking you some questions."

- "Can you tell me your name and age?"
- "Do you know where are you now?"
- "Do you know the date today?"
- Show the patient your pen and ask him, "Do you know what this is?"
- "Now I would like to ask you some questions to check your memory."
- "I will name three objects for you, and I want you to repeat them immediately, okay? Chair, bed, and pen." (Tests immediate memory.)
- "I will ask you to repeat the names of these three objects after a few minutes." (Tests short-term memory.)
- "Do you remember what you had for lunch yesterday?" (Tests recent memory.)
- "When did you get married?" (Tests distant memory.)
- "Now, can you repeat for me the names of the three objects that I mentioned to you?" (Tests short-term memory.)
- "Are you left-handed or right-handed?"
- "I will give you a piece of paper. I want you to take the paper in your right hand, fold the paper in half, and put it on the floor." (Three-step command.)
- "Now I want you to write your name on the paper."
- "I want you to count backward starting with the number 100," or "Take 7 away from 100 and tell me what number you get; then keeping taking 7 away until I tell you to stop." (Tests concentration.)
- "What would you do if you saw a fire coming out from a paper basket?" (Tests judgment.)

- **What to say to the patient before and during the exam—neurologic exam questions:**
  - "I am going to check your reflexes now."
  - "I am going to test the strength of your muscles now."
  - "This is up, and this is down. Tell me which direction I am moving your big toe."
  - "Can you walk across the room for me, please?"
- **What to perform during the neurologic exam:**
  - Mental status examination: Orientation, memory, concentration.
  - Cranial nerves:
    1. II: Vision.
    2. III, IV, VI: Extraocular movements.
    3. V: Facial sensation, muscles of mastication.
    4. VII: Smile, lifting of brows, close your eyes and don't let me open them.
    5. IX, X: Symmetrical palate movement, gag reflex.
    6. XI: Shrug your shoulders.
    7. XII: Stick out your tongue.
  - Motor system:
    1. Passive motion.
    2. Active motion: Arms—flexion (pull in), extension (push out); wrists—flexion (push down), extension (pull up).

3. Hands: Spread your fingers apart, close your fist.
4. Legs: Knee extension (kick out), knee flexion (pull in).
5. Ankles: Push on the gas.

- Reflexes: Biceps, triceps, brachioradialis, patellar, Achilles, Babinski.
- Sensory system: Sharp (pin)/dull (cotton swab), vibration, position sense.
- Cerebellum: Finger-to-nose, heel-to-shin, rapid alternating movements, Romberg sign, gait.
- Meningeal signs: Neck stiffness, Kernig, Brudzinski.

6. Joint exam
   - **What to say to the patient before and during the exam:**
     - "Tell me if you feel pain anywhere."
     - "I am going to examine your knee/ankle now."
   - **What to perform during the joint exam:**
     - Inspect and compare joint with the opposite side.
     - Palpate.
     - Check for joint effusion.
     - Check for crepitus.
     - Check the joint range of motion.

## Special Challenges During the Physical Exam

During the course of the physical exam, you may encounter any number of special problems. The following are examples of such challenges along with potential responses to them.

- **Listening to the heart in a female patient.** You can place the stethoscope anywhere around the patient's bra and between the breasts. To auscultate or palpate the PMI, if necessary, ask the patient, "Can you please lift up your breast?"
- **Examining a patient who is in severe pain.** A patient in severe pain may initially seem unapproachable, refuse the physical exam, and insist that you give him something to stop his pain. In such cases, you should first ask the patient's permission to perform the physical examination. If he refuses, gently say, "I understand that you are in severe pain, and I want to help you. The physical exam that I want to do is very important to help determine what is causing your pain. I will be as quick and gentle as possible, and once I find the reason for your pain, I should be able to give you something to make you more comfortable."
- **Examining lesions.** If you see a scar, a mole (nevus), a psoriatic lesion, or any other skin lesion during the exam, you should mention it and ask the patient about it even if it is not related to the patient's complaint.
- **Examining bruising.** Inquire about any bruises you see on the patient's body, and think about abuse as a possible cause.

## SP Simulation of Physical Exam Findings

It bears repeating that during the physical examination, it is necessary to remain cautious and attentive, as the symptoms patients exhibit during the encounter are seldom accidental and are usually reproducible. So when you notice any positive sign, take it seriously. The following are some physical signs that may be simulated by the SP:

1. Abdomen
   - Abdominal tenderness: The patient feels pain when you press on his abdomen. Remember that the patient is an actor. When you palpate the area, he will feel pain where he is supposed to feel pain regardless of the amount of pressure you exert. So don't try to palpate the same area again; instead, move on, and consider the pain on palpation a positive sign.
   - Abdominal rigidity: The patient will contract his abdominal muscles when you try to palpate the abdomen.
   - Rebound tenderness of the abdomen.
   - CVA tenderness.
2. Chest
   - Shortness of breath.
   - Wheezing: This may often sound strange, as if the patient were whistling from his mouth.
   - Decreased respiratory sounds: The patient will move his chest without really inhaling any air so you do not hear any respiratory sounds.
   - Increased fremitus: The patient will say "99" in a coarse voice, creating more fremitus than usual.
3. Nervous system
   - Confusion.
   - Dementia.
   - Extensor plantar response (Babinski's sign).
   - Absent or hyperactive tendon reflexes (stroke, diabetes mellitus): Eliciting the reflex in the SP is not like doing so in a real patient, where you must try more than once to ensure that you have not missed the tendon and that your strike is strong enough. In a clinical encounter, try the reflex only once; if you don't see it, it is not there. If the patient wants to show you hyperactive DTRs, he will make sure to respond with an exaggerated jerk even to the lightest and most awkward hammer hit.
   - Facial paralysis.
   - Hemiparesis.
   - Gait abnormalities.
   - Ataxia.
   - Chorea.
   - Hearing loss.
   - Tinel's sign.
   - Phalen's sign.

- Nuchal rigidity.
- Kernig's sign.
- Brudzinski's sign.

4. Eyes
   - Visual loss (central, peripheral): In a young patient, this may be multiple sclerosis.
   - Photophobia: The patient will say, "I hate the light" or "I don't feel comfortable in bright light." Dim the light to make the patient feel more comfortable.
   - Lid lag.
   - Nystagmus.

5. Muscles and joints
   - Muscle weakness.
   - Rigidity.
   - Spasticity.
   - Parkinsonism: Shuffling gait (difficulty initiating and stopping ambulation, small steps, no swinging of the arms), resting tremor, masked facies, rare blinking, and cogwheel rigidity.
   - Restricted range of motion of joints.

6. Bruits and murmurs
   - Renal artery stenosis: A patient with hypertension who is not responding to multiple antihypertensive medications. Do not be surprised if you hear an abdominal bruit.
   - Thyroid bruit.
   - Carotid bruit: The patient says "Hush, hush" when you place the stethoscope over his neck.
   - Heart murmur: Once you place the stethoscope on the patient's heart, you will hear him saying "Hush, hush."

7. Skin
   - Skin lesions: You may see artificial skin discoloration (e.g., painful red spots on the shin for erythema nodosum in a patient with sarcoidosis; redness over an inflamed joint in a patient with arthritis).

8. Real physical exam findings
   - You may see real C-section, appendectomy, cholecystectomy, or other scars. Don't overlook them. Always inquire about any scar you see.
   - You may see a real nevus (mole). Ask the patient about it and advise him to check it routinely and report any change in it.
   - You may see real skin lesions, such as pityriasis rosea in a Christmas tree pattern, seborrheic dermatitis of the scalp, or acne vulgaris.
   - When you listen to a patient's heart, don't be surprised to hear a real heart murmur.
   - A patient with a sore throat may present with real enlarged tonsils.

Finishing the history and the physical exam does not mean that the encounter is over. To the contrary, closure is a critical part of the encounter. See Figure 2-4 for an overview of the process. During closure, you are expected to do several things:

- Make a transition to mark the end of your encounter.
- Summarize the chief complaint and the HPI if you have not already done so before the physical examination.
- Summarize your findings from the physical exam.
- Give your impression of the patient's clinical condition and most likely diagnosis.
- Suggest a diagnostic workup.
- Answer any questions the patient might have.
- Address the patient's concerns.
- Check to see if the patient has any more questions.
- Leave the room.

To transition into the closure, you should begin by saying something like "Thank for letting me examine you, Mrs. Jones. Now I would like to sit down with you and give you my impression." You should then tell the patient about the possible differential diagnoses (keep to a maximum of three) and explain the meaning of any complicated medical terms you might use. You might also point out the organ or system that you think is involved and explain a simple mechanism of the disease. You should not, however, give the patient a defini-

*Leave a few minutes for closure. Don't rush it.*

**THE PATIENT ENCOUNTER**

**Figure 2-4. Closure Overview**

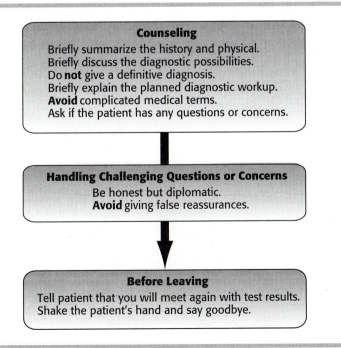

**Counseling**
Briefly summarize the history and physical.
Briefly discuss the diagnostic possibilities.
Do **not** give a definitive diagnosis.
Briefly explain the planned diagnostic workup.
**Avoid** complicated medical terms.
Ask if the patient has any questions or concerns.

**Handling Challenging Questions or Concerns**
Be honest but diplomatic.
**Avoid** giving false reassurances.

**Before Leaving**
Tell patient that you will meet again with test results.
Shake the patient's hand and say goodbye.

tive diagnosis at this time. Instead, tell him that you still need to run some tests in order to establish the final diagnosis. In some cases there will actually be no final diagnosis; instead, the case will be constructed in such a way as to be a mixture of signs and symptoms that can be construed to indicate any number of diseases.

During closure, almost every patient will have at least one challenging question to which you must respond (e.g., " Do you think I have cancer, doctor?" or "Am I going to get better?"). In answering these questions, be honest yet diplomatic. Essentially, being honest with the patient means not giving false reassurances such as "I am sure you will be cured after a week of antibiotics," or "Don't worry, I am sure that it is not cancer." What you might say instead is "Well, I cannot exclude the possibility of cancer at this point. We need to do additional testing. Regardless of the final diagnosis, however, I want you to be assured that I will be available for any support you need."

If you do not know the answer to a patient's question, you should state as much. See the end of this chapter for examples of challenging questions patients might pose along with potential responses to them.

During closure, you should also explain to the patient the diagnostic tests you are planning to order. In doing so, you should again use nontechnical terms— for example, "We need to run some blood tests to check the function of your liver and kidney," or "You need to have a chest x-ray and a CT scan of the head." You may further explain the latter by saying, "The CT scan is a type of x-ray imaging that gives us clear images of sections of the body." You should then add, "After we get the results of those tests, we will meet again to discuss them in detail along with the final diagnosis and the treatment plan." Finally, you should conclude by asking the patient if he still has any questions.

*You cannot reenter the room once you leave.*

Before you leave the room, you can finish your encounter by looking the patient in the eye and saying something like "Okay, Mr. Jones, I'll contact you when I have your test results. It was nice meeting you." You may then shake the patient's hand and leave the room. You are allowed to leave the room as soon as you think you have completed the encounter. Once you have left the encounter room, you will not be allowed to go back inside.

## ▶ HOW TO INTERACT WITH SPECIAL PATIENTS

The following are guidelines for dealing with atypical or uncommon patients.

**The anxious patient.** Encourage the patient to talk about his feelings. Ask him about the things that are causing him to feel anxious. Give him reasonable reassurance.

**The angry patient.** Stay calm and don't be scared. Remember that the patient is not really angry; he is just acting angry to test your response. Let him express his feelings, and ask about the reason for his anger. You should also address the patient's anger in a reasonable way. For example, if the patient is complaining that he has been waiting for a long time, tell him you understand. Explain that the clinic is crowded, and there were many patients who had appointments prior to his. Reassure the patient that now that it is his turn, you will focus on his case and take care of him.

**The crying patient.** Allow the crying patient to express his feelings, and wait in silence for him to finish. Offer him a tissue, and show him empathy in your facial expressions. You may also place your hand lightly on the patient's shoulder or arm and say something like "I know that you feel sad. Would you like to tell me about it?" Don't worry about time constraints in such cases. Remember that the patient is an actor and that his crying is timed. He will allow you to continue the encounter in peace if you respond correctly.

**The patient who is in pain.** Show compassion for the patient's pain. Say something like "I know that you are in pain." Offer help by asking, "Is there anything I can do for you to help you feel more comfortable?" Do not repeat painful maneuvers. If the patient does not allow you to touch his abdomen because of the severe pain he is experiencing, tell him, "I know that you are in pain, and I want to help you. I need to examine you, though, to be able to locate the source of pain and give you the right treatment." Reassure the patient by saying, "I will be as quick and gentle as possible."

**The patient who can't pay for the tests or for treatment.** Reassure the patient by saying, "Not having enough money doesn't mean you can't get treatment." You might also add, "We will refer you to a social worker who can help you find resources."

**The patient who refuses to answer your question or let you examine him.** Explain to the patient why the question or the physical exam is important. Tell him that they are necessary to allow you to understand the problem and arrive at a diagnosis. If the patient still refuses to cooperate, skip the question or the maneuver and document his refusal and your counseling in your PN.

**The hard-of-hearing patient.** Face the patient directly to allow him to read your lips. Speak slowly, and do not cover your mouth. Use gestures to reinforce your words. If the patient has unilateral hearing loss, sit close to the hearing side.

**The patient who doesn't know the names of his medications or is taking medications whose names YOU don't recognize.** Ask the patient if he has a prescription or a written list of the medications he is currently taking.

During your encounters, every patient will ask you one or more challenging questions. Your reaction and answers to these questions will be scored. Such questions may be explicit ones that you are expected to answer directly, or they may take the form of indirect comments or statements that must be properly addressed in order to reveal an underlying concern. When answering the challenging questions, try to remember the following guidelines:

- Be honest and diplomatic.
- Before addressing the patient's issue, you might restate the issue back to the patient to let him know that you understand.
- Don't give the patient a final diagnosis. Instead, tell the patient about your initial impressions and about the workup you have in mind to reach a conclusive diagnosis.
- Do not give false reassurances.
- If you do not know the answer to the patient's question, just tell him so.

The following are examples of challenging questions:

*Do not give the patient a definitive diagnosis.*

## Confidentiality/Ethical Issues

| Challenging Question | Possible Response |
| --- | --- |
| A patient who needs emergent surgery says, "I can't afford the cost of staying in the hospital. I have no insurance. Just give me something to relieve the pain, and I will leave." | "I know that you are concerned about medical costs, but your life will be in danger if you don't have surgery. Let our social workers help you with the cost issues." |
| "Should I tell my sexual partner about my venereal disease?" | "Yes. There is a chance that you have already transmitted the disease to your partner, or he/she may be the source of your infection. The important step is to have you both evaluated and appropriately treated." |
| An anxious patient who you suspect has been abused asks, "Why are you asking me these questions?" | "I am concerned that domestic abuse may be involved. My goal is to make sure that you are in a safe environment and that you are not a victim of abuse." |
| A patient recently diagnosed with HIV asks, "Do I have to tell my wife?" | "I know that it's difficult, but doing so will allow you and your wife to take the appropriate precautions to treat and prevent the transmission of the disease." |

THE PATIENT ENCOUNTER

**Patient Belief/Behavioral Issues**

| Challenging Question | Possible Response |
|---|---|
| An elderly patient says, "I think that it is normal at my age to have this problem" (impotence), or "I am just getting old." | "Age may play a role in the change you are experiencing in your sexual function, but your problem may have other causes that we should rule out, such as certain diseases (hypertension, diabetes) or certain medications. We also have medications that may improve your sexual function." |
| "I read in a journal that the treatment of this disease is herbal compounds." | "Herbal medicines have been suggested for many diseases. However, their safety and efficacy may not always be clear-cut. Let me know the name of the herbal medicine and I will check into its potential treatment role for this disease." |
| "I am afraid of surgery." | "I understand your feelings. It is normal and very common to have these feelings before surgery. Is there anything specific that you are concerned about?" |
| A patient who has a serious problem (unstable angina, colon cancer) asks, "I want to go on a trip with my wife. Can we do the tests after I come back?" | "I know that you don't want to put off your trip, but you may have a serious problem that may benefit from early diagnosis and management." |
| "I did not understand your question, doctor. Could you repeat it, please?" | Repeat the question again slowly. If the patient still doesn't comprehend the question, ask if there is any specific word he didn't understand and try to explain it or use a simpler one. |
| "What is a bronchoscopy?" (MRI, CT, x-ray, colonoscopy) | Explain the meaning using simple words. For example, "Bronchoscopy is using a thin tube connected to a camera to look into your respiratory airways and parts of your lungs," or "An MRI is a machine that uses a big magnet to obtain detailed pictures of your brain or body." |
| "What do you mean by 'workup'?" | "It means all the tests that we are going to do to help us make the final diagnosis." |

| Challenging Question | Possible Response |
|---|---|
| A patient who is late in seeking medical advice asks, "Do you think it is too late for recovery?" | "I am glad that you came for help. We will do our best and hope for the best." |
| A patient with pleuritic chest pain asks, "Is this a heart attack? Am I going to die?" | "Given your current presentation, my suspicion for a heart attack is low. It is more likely that inflammation of the membranes surrounding your lungs is causing your pain, and this is usually not a life-threatening condition. However, we still need to do some tests to confirm the diagnosis and rule out heart problems." |
| "Do you think I have colon cancer?" "Do you think I have a brain tumor?" "Do I have endometrial cancer?" | "That is one of the possibilities, but there are other explanations for your symptoms that we should rule out before making a diagnosis." |
| "My friend told me that you are a very fine doctor. That's why I came to you to refill my prescription." | "I am flattered, but since this is your first visit, I can't give you a refill without reviewing your history to better understand your need for this medication. I will also need to do a physical exam and perhaps order some tests." |
| "Will my insurance cover the expenses of this test?" | "I'm not sure, but I can refer you to a social worker who does have that information. If necessary, I can write a note to your insurance company indicating the importance of this test." |
| A person who wants to return to work at a job that can negatively affect his health asks, "Can I go back to work?" | "Unfortunately, work may actually worsen your condition. Therefore, I prefer that you stay at home for now. I can write a letter to your employer explaining your situation." |
| "Do you think that this tumor I have could become malignant?" | "We really won't know until we remove the mass and get a pathology report on it." |
| "Since I stopped smoking, I have gained weight. I want to go back to smoking in order to lose weight." | "There are healthier ways to lose weight than smoking, such as exercise and diet. Smoking will increase your risk of cancer, heart problems, and lung disease." |

46

| Challenging Question | Possible Response |
|---|---|
| A patient with a shoulder injury says, "I am afraid of losing my job if my shoulder doesn't get better." | "We will do our best to help you recover from your shoulder injury. With your permission, I will communicate the situation to your employer." |
| "Will I ever feel better, doctor?" | The answer differs depending on the prognosis of the disease and can vary from "Yes, most people with this disease are completely cured" to "Complete cure may be difficult at this advanced stage, but we have a lot to offer in terms of controlling the symptoms and improving your quality of life." |
| A person who has a broken arm asks, "Doctor, do you think I will be able to move my arm again like before?" | "It is hard to tell right now, but those fractures usually heal well, and with physical therapy you should regain the normal range of motion of your arm." |
| "I think that life is full of misery. Why do we have to live?" | "Life can be challenging. Is there something in particular that is bothering you? Have you thought of ending your life?" You can then continue screening for depression. |
| A young man with multiple sexual partners and a recent-onset skin rash says, "I am afraid that I might have AIDS." | "Having multiple sexual partners does put you at risk for HIV infection, but this rash may be due to many other causes. I agree that we should do an HIV test on you in addition to a few other tests." |
| A patient who needs hospitalization says, "My child is at home alone. I have to leave now." | "I understand your concern about your child, but right now staying in the hospital is in your best interest. One of our social workers can make some phone calls to arrange for child care." |
| "Do you have anything that will make me feel better? Please, doctor, I am in pain." | "I know that you're in pain, but I need to know what's causing your pain in order to give you the appropriate treatment. After I am done with my evaluation, we can decide on the best way to help manage your pain." |

THE PATIENT ENCOUNTER

| Challenging Question | Possible Response |
|---|---|
| A patient you believe is pretending (malingering) says, "Please, doctor, I need a week off from work. The pain in my back is terrible." | "I know that you are uncomfortable, but after examining you I don't find disability significant enough to keep you out of work. I plan to prescribe pain medication and exercises, but a big part of your recovery will be continuing your normal daily activities." |
| "Stop asking me all these stupid questions and just give me something for this pain." | "I know that you're in pain, but I need to determine the cause of the pain in order to give you the right treatment. After I am done with my evaluation, we will give you appropriate treatment." |
| "So what's the plan, doctor?" | "After we get the results of your tests, we will meet again. At that time, I will try to answer any questions you may have." |
| "Do you think I will need surgery?" | "I will try to manage your problem medically, but if that doesn't work, you may need surgery. We can see how things go and then try to make that decision together in the future." |
| A female patient has only one partner, and she is diagnosed with an STD. She asks you, "Could he possibly be cheating on me?" | "You most likely contracted this infection from your partner. It would be best to talk to your partner about this to clear things up. He needs to be tested and treated, or else you risk becoming reinfected." |
| A patient is shouting angrily, "Where have you been, doctor? I have been waiting here for the whole day." | "I am sorry you had to wait so long. We had some unexpected delays with a few of the earlier patients this morning. But I'm here now, and I will focus on you and your concerns." |

**Disease-Related Issues**

| Challenging Question | Possible Response |
|---|---|
| An educated 58-year-old woman asks, "I read in a scientific journal that hormonal replacement therapy causes breast cancer. What do you think of that, doctor?" | "It appears to be true. Studies show a slight increase in the risk of developing breast cancer after four years of combination estrogen and progesterone use for hormonal replacement therapy. The current recommendations are to use hormonal replacement therapy solely for the relief of hot flashes and only for a limited period of time." |
| "Do I have a stroke?" | "We don't know yet. Your symptoms could be explained by a small stroke, but we need to wait for the results of your MRI." |
| "Do I have lung cancer?" | "We don't know at this point. It could be a possibility, but we still need to do additional tests." |
| An African-American male with sickle cell anemia presents with back and chest pain and says, "Please, doctor, I need some Demerol now or I will die from pain." | "I know that you are in pain, but I need to ask you a few questions first to better understand your pain. Then we will get you medicines for your pain." |
| A patient with symptoms of a common cold says, "I think I need antibiotics, doctor." | "It appears that you have a viral common cold. Antibiotics do not treat viruses, and they have side effects that could even make you feel worse. We should focus on treating your symptoms." |
| "My mother had breast cancer. What is the possibility that I will have breast cancer too?" | "You are at increased risk, but it doesn't mean that you will get it. There are other risk factors that need to be considered, and regular screening tests will be very important." |
| A 55-year-old male says, "I had a colonoscopy six years ago, and they removed a polyp. Do you think that I have to repeat the colonoscopy?" | "Yes, it should be repeated. We need to screen for more polyps, and in this way we hope to prevent the development of colon cancer." |

| Challenging Question | Possible Response |
|---|---|
| A patient with headache or confusion asks, "Do you think I have Alzheimer's disease?" | "I don't know. Alzheimer's is one of several possible causes that we will investigate." |
| "Can I get pregnant even though my tubes are tied?" | "There is no single contraceptive method that is 100% effective. The risk of pregnancy after tubal ligation is less than 1%, but it is a real risk." |
| A woman who is in her first trimester of pregnancy with vaginal bleeding asks, "Do you think I am losing my pregnancy?" | "Bleeding early in pregnancy increases your risk of losing the pregnancy, but at the same time, most women who have bleeding carry the pregnancy to term without problems." |
| "My brother has colon cancer. What are the chances that I will have colon cancer as well?" | "Some types of colon cancer are hereditary, and you may be at increased risk, but it doesn't mean that you will get colon cancer for sure. I need to get more information about your personal and family history to determine your level of risk." |
| A patient with palpitations says, "My mother had a thyroid problem; do you think it is my thyroid?" | "It's possible. We always check a thyroid blood test, but we will also consider many other possible causes of palpitations." |
| "Obesity runs in my family. Do you think that this is why I am overweight?" | "Genes play an important role in obesity, but lifestyle, diet, and daily habits are also major factors influencing weight. These factors can be used in a way that can help you lose weight." |
| A young man with dysuria asks, "Do you think I have an STD?" | "That is one of the possibilities. We will do some cultures to find out for sure, and we will also check a urine sample, since your symptoms may be due to a urinary tract infection." |
| "I am drinking a lot of water, doctor. What do you think the reason is?" | "This may simply be due to dehydration, or it may be a sign of a disease such as diabetes. We need to do some tests to determine the cause." |

| Challenging Question | Possible Response |
| --- | --- |
| A patient with COPD asks, "Will I get better if I stop smoking?" | "Most patients with your condition who stop smoking will experience a gradual improvement in their symptoms, in addition to the significantly decreased risk of lung cancer in the future." |
| A patient with possible appendicitis is asking for a cup of water to drink. | "I am sorry, but I can't give you anything to eat or drink right now. You may need emergent surgery, and anesthesia is much safer if your stomach is completely empty." |
| A patient with infectious mononucleosis asks, "Can I go back to school, doctor?" | "Now that you have recovered from the acute stage of the disease, you can go back to school, but I want you to stay away from any strenuous exercise or contact sports, as you may rupture your spleen." |

▶ THE PATIENT NOTE

Once you have completed an encounter, your final task will be to compose a PN. (See Figure 2-5 for a detailed overview of the clinical encounter and PN.) Toward this goal, you will find a desk with a sheet of paper on it immediately outside the encounter room. You will be given 10 minutes to write the PN and will be notified when two minutes remain. If you leave the encounter room before the end of the 15-minute period allotted for your patient encounter, you can devote the extra time you have to writing the PN. You are allowed to review the doorway information while you are writing the PN.

The PN sheet located outside the encounter room will have your name, the number of the encounter, and a bar code printed on it. You will not be provided with additional paper, so use the space wisely. You should also take care not to write outside the frame of the sheet, because the paper will be scanned and nothing outside the frame will be read. Be sure to use the pen provided by the examination center, as you are not allowed to use your own pens.

Before you start writing the PN, take a few seconds to review the history, including the chief complaint, how it started, its progression, and the main symptoms. Then take a deep breath and try to relax. If you get nervous and try to rush, your thoughts may become garbled, and you will risk losing the point of your story. As you begin to write, also remember that your handwriting must be legible in order for your PN to be properly scored.

Figure 2-5. Summary Overview of the Patient Encounter

**THE PATIENT ENCOUNTER**

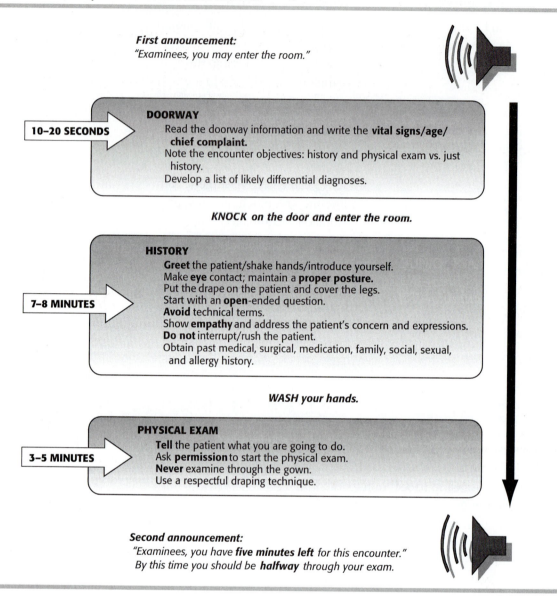

*First announcement:*
*"Examinees, you may enter the room."*

**10–20 SECONDS**

**DOORWAY**
Read the doorway information and write the **vital signs/age/ chief complaint.**
Note the encounter objectives: history and physical exam vs. just history.
Develop a list of likely differential diagnoses.

*KNOCK on the door and enter the room.*

**7–8 MINUTES**

**HISTORY**
**Greet** the patient/shake hands/introduce yourself.
Make **eye** contact; maintain a **proper posture.**
Put the drape on the patient and cover the legs.
Start with an **open**-ended question.
**Avoid** technical terms.
Show **empathy** and address the patient's concern and expressions.
**Do not** interrupt/rush the patient.
Obtain past medical, surgical, medication, family, social, sexual, and allergy history.

*WASH your hands.*

**3–5 MINUTES**

**PHYSICAL EXAM**
**Tell** the patient what you are going to do.
Ask **permission** to start the physical exam.
**Never** examine through the gown.
Use a respectful draping technique.

*Second announcement:*
*"Examinees, you have **five minutes left** for this encounter."*
*By this time you should be **halfway** through your exam.*

## Writing the Patient Note

You will be required to fill out four main sections in your PN: the history, physical exam, differential diagnosis, and initial diagnostic workup.

**Summarizing the history.** In writing the history, be clear, direct, and concise, and avoid long and complex phrases. Make sure the history flows in a logical order. Also bear in mind that it is not necessary to write a detailed, all-inclusive history. The components that should be included are as follows:

- Chief complaint (CC)
- History of present illness (HPI)
- Review of systems (ROS)
- Past medical history (PMH)
- Past surgical history (PSH)

Figure 2-5. **Summary Overview of the Patient Encounter** *(continued)*

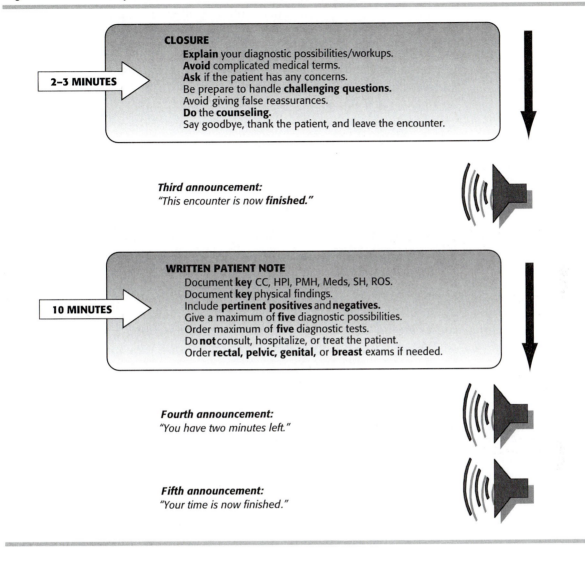

- Social history (SH)
- Family history (FH)

When you are summarizing the history, you should be prudent in using the space assigned to you for that purpose. Many examinees run out of space while writing this section. One way to save both time and space is to make ample use of abbreviations. Train yourself to use the abbreviations that are listed in the USMLE Step 2 CS exam orientation materials (Please see inside back cover). You will find a copy of this list on each desk. You are allowed to use any abbreviations that are commonly used in U.S. hospitals. If you are unsure of the correct abbreviation, it is better to spell out the word.

In general, many different styles of writing are acceptable as long as your history is both comprehensive and legible. Two examples can be found in the candidate orientation manual.

**Outlining the physical exam.** To summarize the physical exam, write a list of the systems that you examined, outlining all the relevant positive and negative findings. If you did not perform a maneuver that you think was necessary, it is better not to lie and pretend that you did. Be honest and list only the items you examined. For example, do not claim that you saw diabetic retinopathy in a patient with diabetes mellitus if you did not even get to see the eye fundus. See Figure 2-6 for some examples of how to document physical exam findings.

**Developing a differential.** In writing the differential, you should list a maximum of five diagnoses. You are not required to list that many if three or four diagnoses suffice. The diagnoses should be directly related to the history and physical exam, and it is preferable that they be listed in order of probability, from the most to the least probable.

**Specifying the initial diagnostic workup.** In summarizing your workup, list a maximum of five tests. It is best to start with the "forbidden physical examination maneuvers" (e.g., rectal exam, pelvic exam) if you feel such procedures are indicated. Then state the required laboratory and radiologic tests, starting with the most simple and straightforward tests and ending with the most complex. Do not include referrals, treatments, hospitalizations, or consults, as these will not be scored.

*Tests in the diagnostic workup should be specific.*

Be specific in your orders. Instead of "chem 7," "thyroid panel," or "liver function tests," you should specify "Na, K," "TSH and total $T_4$," and "AST and ALT." You may, however, order electrolytes. Each group of related tests (blood tests, x-rays) should be listed together.

### Scoring the Patient Note

The PN will be scored by a physician on the basis of its organization, quality of information, interpretation of data, and legibility. The final score will represent the average PN score of all 10 scored encounters.

### How to Prepare

The cardinal rule for preparing to write a PN is to practice, practice, and practice. Imagine that you are in the actual exam and try to write the PN within 10 minutes. You should also practice writing the note so that it will fit in the allotted space. When using the cases presented in this book, try to write your PN and then compare your note with ours. The main things you should look for are the following:

- Is your history complete?
- Does it make sense?
- Are the physical exam results complete?

Figure 2-6. Examples of How to Document Physical Exam Findings

- **HEENT:**
  - Head: Atraumatic, normocephalic.
  - Eyes: EOMI, PERRLA, normal eye fundus.
  - Nose: No nasal congestion.
  - Throat: No tonsillar erythema, exudates, or enlargement.
  - Mouth: Moist mucous membranes, good dentition, no lesions.

- **Neck:** Supple, no JVD, normal thyroid, no cervical LAD.

- **Nervous System:**
  - Mental status: Alert and oriented x 3, good concentration.
  - Cranial nerves II–XII grossly intact.
  - Motor: Strength 5/5 in all muscle groups.
  - DTRs: 2+ intact and symmetric, Babinski ⊖.
  - Sensation: Intact to sharp and dull.
  - Cerebellum: ⊖ Romberg sign, intact finger to nose.

- **Chest/Lung:**
  - Clear to percussion bilaterally.
  - No rales, rhonchi, wheezing, or rubs.
  - No tenderness to palpation.
  - Tactile fremitus WNL.

- **Heart:**
  - PMI not displaced.
  - Regular rate and rhythm.
  - Normal S1, S2.
  - No murmurs, rubs, or gallops.

- **Abdomen:**
  - Soft, nontender, nondistended, BS ⊕, no hepatosplenomegaly.

- **Extremities:**
  - No clubbing, cyanosis, or edema.

- **Mental Status Exam:**
  - Patient speaks slowly.
  - No hostile behavior toward the interviewer.
  - Blunt affect with poor eye contact.
  - Inattentive to interviewer.
  - 3/3 registration, 3/3 recall at 3 times.
  - Distant memories are impaired.
  - Oriented to person, date, and place.
  - Completed three-step command.
  - Right-handed.
  - 1/5 on serial 7s.
  - Poor judgment.

THE PATIENT ENCOUNTER

- Is your differential diagnosis correct?
- Are your tests correct and in the right order?

There are several styles you can use both to document the physical exam and to compose the PN. So choose a method, memorize it, and stick with it. Note, however, that in this book we used only one method to write PNs.

# SECTION III

# Minicases

In this chapter, we will attempt to cover most of the clinical cases that you are likely to encounter in the Step 2 CS. The main title of each case represents a chief complaint that you may see on the doorway information sheet before you enter the examination room. After each chief complaint, key points pertinent to the history and physical exam are reviewed. Each clinical case consists of three components:

- **Presentation:** A brief clinical case with some pertinent positives and negatives.
- **Differential:** An appropriate differential diagnosis, with the most likely diagnosis appearing in boldface.
- **Workup:** The main diagnostic tests that should be considered for each disease. Note that the diagnostic tests in the third column are generally listed in order of priority. In clinical practice, many tests may be performed at the same time or not at all.

The sum of the **Differential** column will give you a wide differential diagnosis for the chief complaint, while the sum of the **Workup** column will give you a pool of tests from which to choose in the exam.

If you are studying by yourself, we suggest that you start by reading the vignette and then try to figure out the diagnosis and the workup.

If you are studying with a partner or in a group, we suggest that you read a vignette aloud and have others develop the differential diagnosis and workup.

## Key History

Location (especially unilateral vs. bilateral), quality, intensity, duration, timing (does it disturb sleep?); presence of associated neurologic symptoms, nausea, jaw claudication; recent trauma, dental surgery, sinusitis symptoms; exacerbating (stress, fatigue, menses, exercise) and alleviating factors (rest, medicines); past history of headache; family history of migraines.

## Key Physical Exam

Vital signs; inspection and palpation of entire head; ENT inspection; complete neurologic exam, including funduscopic exam.

| Presentation | Differential | Workup |
|---|---|---|
| 21 yo F presents with several episodes of throbbing left temporal pain that lasts for 2–3 hours. Prior to its onset, she sees flashes of light in her right visual field and feels weakness and numbness on the right side of her body for a few minutes. Headaches are often associated with nausea and vomiting. She has a family history of migraine. | **Migraine (complicated)** <br> Tension headache <br> Cluster headache <br> Pseudotumor cerebri <br> Trigeminal neuralgia <br> CNS vasculitis <br> Partial seizure <br> Intracranial neoplasm | CBC <br> ESR <br> CT—head <br> MRI—brain <br> LP |
| 26 yo M presents with terrible right temporal headaches associated with ipsilateral rhinorrhea and eye tearing and redness. Episodes have occurred at the same time every night for the past week and last for 45 minutes. | **Cluster headache** <br> Migraine <br> Tension headache <br> Sinusitis <br> Pseudotumor cerebri <br> Trigeminal neuralgia <br> Intracranial neoplasm | CBC <br> ESR <br> CT—head <br> MRI—brain <br> LP |
| 65 yo F presents with severe, intermittent right temporal headache, fever, blurred vision in her right eye, and pain in her jaw when chewing. | **Temporal arteritis (giant cell arteritis)** <br> Migraine <br> Cluster headache <br> Tension headache <br> Meningitis <br> Carotid artery dissection <br> Pseudotumor cerebri <br> Trigeminal neuralgia <br> Intracranial neoplasm | CBC <br> ESR <br> CRP <br> Temporal artery biopsy <br> Doppler U/S—carotid <br> MRI—brain |

MINICASES

| Presentation | Differential | Workup |
|---|---|---|
| ▪ 30 yo F presents with frontal headache, fever, and nasal discharge. There is pain on palpation of the frontal and maxillary sinuses. She has a history of sinusitis. | **Sinusitis**<br>Migraine<br>Tension headache<br>Meningitis<br>Intracranial neoplasm | CBC<br>CT—sinus<br>LP |
| ▪ 50 yo F presents with recurrent episodes of bilateral squeezing headaches that occur 3–4 times a week. She is experiencing significant stress in her life. | **Tension headache**<br>Migraine<br>Depression<br>Caffeine or analgesic withdrawal<br>Hypertension<br>Cluster headache<br>Pseudotumor cerebri<br>Intracranial neoplasm | CBC<br>Electrolytes<br>ESR<br>CT—head<br>LP |
| ▪ 35 yo M presents with sudden severe headache, vomiting, confusion, left hemiplegia, and nuchal rigidity. | **Subarachnoid hemorrhage**<br>Migraine<br>Meningitis/encephalitis<br>Intracranial hemorrhage<br>Vertebral artery dissection<br>Intracranial venous thrombosis<br>Acute hypertension<br>Intracranial neoplasm | CT—head<br>LP<br>CBC<br>PT/PTT<br>MRI/MRA—brain |
| ▪ 25 yo M presents with high fever, severe headache, confusion, photophobia, and nuchal rigidity. Kernig's and Brudzinski's signs are positive. | **Meningitis**<br>Migraine<br>Subarachnoid hemorrhage<br>Sinusitis/encephalitis<br>Intracranial or epidural abscess | CBC<br>CT—head<br>MRI—brain<br>LP—CSF analysis (cell count, protein, glucose, Gram stain, PCR for antigens, culture) |
| ▪ 18 yo obese F presents with headache, vomiting, and blurred vision for the past 2–3 weeks. She is taking OCPs. | **Pseudotumor cerebri**<br>Tension headache<br>Migraine<br>Cluster headache<br>Meningitis<br>Intracranial venous thrombosis<br>Intracranial neoplasm | Urine hCG<br>CBC<br>CT—head<br>LP—opening pressure and CSF analysis |

| Presentation | Differential | Workup |
|---|---|---|
| 47 yo M c/o daily pain in the right cheek over the past month. The pain is electric in character and occurs while he is shaving. Each episode lasts 2–4 minutes. | **Trigeminal neuralgia**<br>Tension headache<br>Migraine<br>Cluster headache<br>TMJ dysfunction<br>Intracranial neoplasm | CBC<br>ESR<br>MRI—brain |

▶ CONFUSION/MEMORY LOSS

## Key History

Must include history from family members/caregivers. Detailed time course of cognitive deficits, associated symptoms (constitutional, incontinence, ataxia, hypothyroid symptoms, depression); screen for delirium (waxing/waning level of alertness); ADL/IADL status, falls, medications (and recent medication changes); history of stroke or other atherosclerotic vascular disease, syphilis, HIV risk factors, alcohol use, or vitamin $B_{12}$ deficiency; family history of Alzheimer's disease.

## Key Physical Exam

Vital signs; complete neurologic exam, including mini-mental status exam and gait; general physical exam, including ENT, heart, lungs, abdomen, and extremities.

| Presentation | Differential | Workup |
|---|---|---|
| 81 yo M presents with progressive confusion over the past several years together with forgetfulness and clumsiness. He has a history of hypertension, diabetes mellitus, and two strokes with residual left hemiparesis. Mental status has clearly worsened after each stroke. | **Vascular ("multi-infarct")**<br>**dementia**<br>Alzheimer's disease<br>Normal pressure hydrocephalus<br>Chronic subdural hematoma<br>Intracranial tumor<br>Depression<br>$B_{12}$ deficiency<br>Neurosyphilis<br>Hypothyroidism | CBC<br>VDRL/RPR<br>Serum $B_{12}$<br>TSH<br>MRI—brain<br>CT—head<br>LP—CSF analysis (rare) |

| Presentation | Differential | Workup |
|---|---|---|
| 84 yo F brought by her son c/o forgetfulness (e.g., forgets phone numbers, loses her way back home) along with difficulty performing some of her daily activities (e.g., bathing, dressing, managing money, using the phone). The problem has gradually progressed over the past few years. | **Alzheimer's disease**<br>Vascular dementia<br>Depression<br>Hypothyroidism<br>Chronic subdural hematoma<br>Normal pressure hydrocephalus<br>Intracranial tumor<br>$B_{12}$ deficiency<br>Neurosyphilis | CBC<br>VDRL/RPR<br>Serum $B_{12}$<br>TSH<br>MRI—brain (preferred)<br>CT—head<br>LP—CSF analysis (rare) |
| 72 yo M presents with memory loss, gait disturbance, and urinary incontinence for the past six months. | **Normal pressure hydrocephalus**<br>Alzheimer's disease<br>Vascular dementia<br>Chronic subdural hematoma<br>Intracranial tumor<br>Depression<br>$B_{12}$ deficiency<br>Neurosyphilis<br>Hypothyroidism | CT—head<br>LP—opening pressure and CSF analysis<br>Serum $B_{12}$<br>VDRL/RPR<br>TSH |
| 55 yo M presents with a rapidly progressive change in mental status, inability to concentrate, and memory impairment for the past two months. His symptoms are associated with myoclonus and ataxia. | **Creutzfeldt-Jakob disease**<br>Vascular dementia<br>Lewy body dementia<br>Wernicke's encephalopathy<br>Normal pressure hydrocephalus<br>Chronic subdural hematoma<br>Intracranial tumor<br>Depression<br>Delirium<br>$B_{12}$ deficiency<br>Neurosyphilis | CBC, electrolytes, calcium<br>Serum $B_{12}$<br>VDRL/RPR<br>MRI—brain (preferred)<br>CT—head<br>EEG<br>LP—CSF analysis<br>Brain biopsy |
| 70 yo insulin-dependent diabetic M presents with episodes of confusion, dizziness, palpitation, diaphoresis, and weakness. | **Hypoglycemia**<br>Transient ischemic attack<br>Arrhythmia<br>Delirium<br>Angina | Glucose<br>CBC, electrolytes<br>Echocardiography<br>ECG<br>MRI—brain<br>Doppler U/S—carotid |
| 55 yo F presents with gradual altered mental status and headache. Two weeks ago she slipped, hit her head on the ground, and lost consciousness for two minutes. | **Subdural hematoma**<br>SIADH (causing hyponatremia)<br>Creutzfeldt-Jakob disease<br>Intracranial tumor | Electrolytes<br>CT—head<br>MRI—brain<br>LP |

MINICASES

## Key History

Lightheadedness vs. vertigo, ± auditory symptoms (hearing loss, tinnitus), duration of episodes, context (occurs with positioning, following head trauma), other associated symptoms (visual disturbance, URI, nausea); neck pain or injury; medications; history of atherosclerotic vascular disease.

## Key Physical Exam

Vital signs; complete neurologic exam, including Romberg test, nystagmus, tilt test (e.g., Dix-Hallpike maneuver), gait, hearing, and Weber and Rinne tests; head and neck exam; cardiovascular exam.

| Presentation | Differential | Workup |
|---|---|---|
| 35 yo F presents with intermittent episodes of vertigo, tinnitus, nausea, and hearing loss over the past week. | **Ménière's disease**<br>Vestibular neuronitis<br>Labyrinthitis<br>Benign positional vertigo<br>Acoustic neuroma | CBC<br>VDRL/RPR (syphilis is a cause of Ménière's disease)<br>MRI—brain |
| 55 yo F c/o dizziness for the past day. She feels faint and has severe diarrhea that started two days ago. She takes furosemide for her hypertension. | **Orthostatic hypotension due to dehydration** (diarrhea, diuretic use)<br>Vestibular neuronitis<br>Labyrinthitis<br>Benign positional vertigo<br>Vertebrobasilar insufficiency | Orthostatic vital signs<br>CBC<br>Electrolytes<br>Stool exam (occult blood, fecal leukocytes) |
| 65 yo M presents with postural dizziness and unsteadiness. He has hypertension and was started on hydrochlorothiazide two days ago. | **Drug-induced orthostatic hypotension**<br>Vestibular neuronitis<br>Labyrinthitis<br>Benign positional vertigo<br>Brain stem or cerebellar tumor<br>Acute renal failure | Orthostatic vital signs<br>CBC<br>Electrolytes<br>BUN/Cr<br>MRI—brain |
| 44 yo F c/o dizziness on moving her head to the left. She feels that the room is spinning around her head. Tilt test results in nystagmus and nausea. | **Benign positional vertigo**<br>Vestibular neuronitis<br>Labyrinthitis<br>Ménière's disease | MRI—brain<br>Audiogram |

| Presentation | Differential | Workup |
|---|---|---|
| 55 yo F c/o dizziness that started this morning. She is nauseated and has vomited once in the past day. She had a URI two days ago and has experienced no hearing loss. | **Vestibular neuronitis**<br>Labyrinthitis<br>Ménière's disease<br>Benign positional vertigo<br>Vertigo associated with cervical spine disease/injury<br>Vertebrobasilar insufficiency | CBC<br>Electrolytes<br>Electronystagmography<br>MRI/MRA—brain |
| 55 yo F c/o dizziness that started this morning and of "not hearing well." She feels nauseated and has vomited once in the past day. She had a URI two days ago. | **Labyrinthitis**<br>Vestibular neuronitis<br>Ménière's disease<br>Acoustic neuroma<br>Vertebrobasilar insufficiency | Audiogram<br>Electronystagmography<br>MRI/MRA—brain |

► **LOSS OF CONSCIOUSNESS (LOC)**

## Key History

Presence or absence of preceding symptoms (nausea, diaphoresis, palpitation, pallor, lightheadedness), context (exertional, postural, traumatic; stressful, painful, or claustrophobic experience; dehydration); associated tongue biting, incontinence, tonic-clonic movements, prolonged confusion; dyspnea or pulmonary embolism risk factors; history of heart disease or arrhythmia; alcohol and drug use.

## Key Physical Exam

Vital signs, including orthostatics; complete neurologic exam; carotid and cardiac exam; lung exam.

| Presentation | Differential | Workup |
|---|---|---|
| 26 yo M presents after falling and losing consciousness at work. He had rhythmic movements of the limbs, bit his tongue, and lost control of his bladder. He was subsequently confused (as witnessed by his colleagues). | **Seizure, grand mal** (now called complex tonic-clonic seizure)<br>Convulsive syncope<br>Substance abuse/overdose<br>Malingering<br>Hypoglycemia | CBC, electrolytes, glucose<br>Urine toxicology<br>EEG<br>MRI—brain<br>CT—head<br>LP—CSF analysis<br>ECG |

| Presentation | Differential | Workup |
|---|---|---|
| ▪ 55 yo M c/o falling after feeling dizzy and unsteady. He experienced transient LOC. He has hypertension and is on numerous antihypertensive drugs. | **Drug-induced orthostatic hypotension (causing syncope)** <br> Cardiac arrhythmia <br> Syncope (vasovagal, other causes) <br> Stroke <br> MI <br> Pulmonary embolism | Orthostatic vital signs <br> CBC <br> Electrolytes <br> CT—head <br> ECG <br> V/Q scan <br> CT—chest with IV contrast |
| ▪ 65 yo M presents after falling and losing consciousness for a few seconds. He had no warning prior to passing out but recently had palpitations. His past history includes coronary artery bypass grafting (CABG). | **Cardiac arrhythmia (causing syncope)** <br> Severe aortic stenosis <br> Syncope (other causes) <br> Seizure <br> Pulmonary embolism | ECG <br> Holter monitoring <br> CBC, electrolytes <br> Glucose <br> Echocardiography <br> CT—head |

▶ **NUMBNESS/WEAKNESS**

### Key History

Distribution (unilateral, bilateral, proximal, distal), duration, ± progressive, pain (especially headache, neck or back pain); constitutional symptoms, other neurologic symptoms; history of diabetes, alcoholism, atherosclerotic vascular disease.

### Key Physical Exam

Vital signs; neurologic and musculoskeletal exams; relevant vascular exam.

| Presentation | Differential | Workup |
|---|---|---|
| ▪ 68 yo M presents following a 20-minute episode of slurred speech, right facial drooping and numbness, and right hand weakness. His symptoms had totally resolved by the time he got to the ER. He has a history of hypertension, diabetes mellitus, and heavy smoking. | **Transient ischemic attack (TIA)** <br> Hypoglycemia <br> Seizure | CBC <br> Glucose <br> Electrolytes <br> ECG <br> CT—head <br> MRI—brain <br> Doppler U/S—carotid <br> Echocardiography <br> EEG |

| Presentation | Differential | Workup |
|---|---|---|
| 68 yo M presents with slurred speech, right facial drooping and numbness, and right hand weakness. Babinski's sign is present on the right. He has a history of hypertension, diabetes mellitus, and heavy smoking. | **Stroke**<br>TIA<br>Seizure<br>Intracranial tumor<br>Subdural or epidural hematoma | CBC, electrolytes<br>PT/PTT<br>CT—head<br>MRI—brain (preferred)<br>Doppler U/S—carotid<br>Echocardiography |
| 33 yo F presents with ascending loss of strength in her lower legs over the past two weeks. She had a recent URI. | **Guillain-Barré syndrome**<br>Multiple sclerosis<br>Polymyositis<br>Myasthenia gravis<br>Peripheral neuropathy<br>Tumor in the vertebral canal | CBC, electrolytes<br>CPK<br>LP—CSF analysis<br>MRI—spine<br>EMG/nerve conduction study<br>Serum $B_{12}$ |
| 30 yo F presents with weakness, loss of sensation, and tingling in her left leg that started this morning. She is also experiencing right eye pain, decreased vision, and double vision. She reports feeling "electric shocks" down her spine upon flexing her head. | **Multiple sclerosis**<br>Stroke<br>Conversion disorder<br>Malingering<br>CNS tumor<br>Neurosyphilis<br>Syringomyelia<br>CNS vasculitis | CBC, ESR<br>RPR/VDRL<br>MRI—brain<br>LP—CSF analysis<br>Retinal evoked potentials |
| 55 yo M presents with tingling and numbness in the hands and feet (glove and stocking distribution) over the past two months. He has a history of diabetes mellitus, hypertension, and alcoholism. There is decreased soft touch, vibratory, and position sense in the feet. | **Diabetic peripheral neuropathy**<br>Alcoholic peripheral neuropathy<br>$B_{12}$ deficiency<br>Hypocalcemia<br>Hyperventilation<br>Paraproteinemia/myeloma | ESR<br>Calcium<br>Serum $B_{12}$<br>Glucose, hemoglobin $A_{1c}$<br>  ($HgA_{1c}$)<br>SPEP/UPEP |
| 40 yo F presents with occasional double vision and droopy eyelids at night with normalization by morning. | **Myasthenia gravis**<br>Horner's syndrome<br>Multiple sclerosis<br>Intracranial tumor compressing CN III, IV, or VI<br>Amyotrophic lateral sclerosis | Tensilon test<br>ACh receptor antibodies (in serum)<br>CXR<br>CT—chest<br>MRI—brain<br>EMG |

| Presentation | Differential | Workup |
|---|---|---|
| 25 yo M presents with hemiparesis (after a tonic-clonic seizure) that resolves over a few hours. | **Todd's paralysis**<br>TIA<br>Stroke<br>Complicated migraine<br>Malingering | CBC, electrolytes<br>EEG<br>MRI—brain<br>Doppler U/S—carotid |

## Key History

Duration; sleep hygiene, snoring, waking up choking/gasping, witnessed apnea; overexertion; stress, depression, or other emotional problems; diet; weight changes; other constitutional symptoms; symptoms of thyroid disease; history of bleeding or anemia; medications; alcohol and drug use.

## Key Physical Exam

Vital signs; head and neck exam (conjunctival pallor, oropharynx/palate, lymphadenopathy, thyroid exam); heart, lung, abdominal, and neurologic exams; consider rectal exam and occult blood testing.

| Presentation | Differential | Workup |
|---|---|---|
| 40 yo F c/o feeling tired, hopeless, and worthless and of having suicidal thoughts. She recently discovered that her husband is gay. | **Depression**<br>Adjustment disorder<br>Hypothyroidism<br>Anemia | CBC<br>TSH<br>HIV/STD testing (given husband's possible risk factors) |
| 44 yo M presents with fatigue, insomnia, and nightmares about a murder that he witnessed in a mall one year ago. Since then, he has avoided that mall and has not gone out at night. | **Post-traumatic stress disorder (PTSD)**<br>Depression<br>Generalized anxiety disorder<br>Psychotic or delusional disorder<br>Hypothyroidism | CBC<br>TSH<br>Calcium<br>Urine toxicology |
| 55 yo M presents with fatigue, weight loss, and constipation. He has a family history of colon cancer. | **Colon cancer**<br>Hypothyroidism<br>Renal failure<br>Hypercalcemia<br>Other malignancy<br>Depression | Rectal exam, stool for occult blood<br>CBC, electrolytes, calcium, BUN/Cr, AST/ALT, TSH<br>Colonoscopy<br>Barium enema |

| Presentation | Differential | Workup |
|---|---|---|
| 40 yo F presents with fatigue, weight gain, sleepiness, cold intolerance, constipation, and dry skin. | **Hypothyroidism** <br> Depression <br> Diabetes <br> Anemia | TSH <br> CBC <br> Glucose |
| 50 yo obese F presents with fatigue and daytime sleepiness. She snores heavily and naps 3–4 times per day but never feels refreshed. She also has hypertension. | **Obstructive sleep apnea** <br> Hypothyroidism <br> Chronic fatigue syndrome | CBC <br> TSH <br> Nocturnal pulse oximetry <br> Polysomnography <br> ECG |
| 20 yo M presents with fatigue, thirst, increased appetite, and polyuria. | **Diabetes mellitus** <br> Atypical depression <br> Primary polydipsia <br> Diabetes insipidus | Glucose <br> UA <br> CBC, electrolytes <br> BUN/Cr |
| 35 yo M policeman c/o feeling tired and sleepy during the day. He changed to the night shift last week. | **Sleep deprivation** <br> Sleep apnea <br> Depression <br> Anemia | CBC <br> Nocturnal pulse oximetry <br> Polysomnography |

► **SORE THROAT**

**Key History**

Duration, fever, other ENT symptoms (ear pain, URI), odynophagia, swollen glands, ± cough, rash; sick contacts, HIV risk factors.

**Key Physical Exam**

Vital signs; ENT exam, including oral thrush, tonsillar exudate, and lymphadenopathy; lung, abdominal, and skin exams.

| Presentation | Differential | Workup |
|---|---|---|
| 26 yo F presents with sore throat, fever, severe fatigue, and loss of appetite for the past week. She also reports epigastric and LUQ discomfort. She has cervical lymphadenopathy and a rash. Her boyfriend recently experienced similar symptoms. | **Infectious mononucleosis** <br> Hepatitis <br> Viral or bacterial pharyngitis <br> Acute HIV infection <br> Secondary syphilis | CBC, peripheral smear <br> Monospot test <br> Throat culture <br> AST/ALT/bilirubin/alkaline phosphatase <br> HIV antibody and viral load <br> Anti-EBV antibodies <br> VDRL/RPR |

| Presentation | Differential | Workup |
|---|---|---|
| 26 yo M presents with sore throat, fever, rash, and weight loss. He has a history of IV drug abuse and sharing needles. | **HIV, acute retroviral syndrome** Infectious mononucleosis Hepatitis Viral pharyngitis Streptococcal tonsillitis/scarlet fever Secondary syphilis | CBC Peripheral smear HIV antibody and viral load CD4 count Monospot test Throat culture VDRL/RPR AST/ALT/bilirubin/alkaline phosphatase |
| 26 yo F presents with fever and sore throat. | **Pharyngitis (bacterial or viral)** *Mycoplasma* pneumonia Acute HIV infection Infectious mononucleosis | Throat swab for culture and rapid streptococcal antigen Monospot test CBC HIV antibody and viral load |

▶ **COUGH/SHORTNESS OF BREATH**

**Key History**

Acute vs. chronic; presence/description of sputum, associated symptoms (constitutional, URI, postnasal drip, dyspnea, wheezing, chest pain, heartburn, other), exacerbating and alleviating factors; exposures; smoking history; history of lung disease; allergies; medicines (especially ACE inhibitors).

**Key Physical Exam**

Vital signs ± pulse oximetry; exam of nasal mucosa, oropharynx, heart, lungs, lymph nodes, and extremities (clubbing, cyanosis, edema).

| Presentation | Differential | Workup |
|---|---|---|
| 30 yo M presents with shortness of breath, cough, and wheezing that worsen in cold air. He has had several such episodes over the past four months. | **Asthma** GERD Bronchitis Pneumonitis Foreign body CBC | CXR Peak flow measurement PFTs Methacholine challenge test |
| 56 yo F presents with shortness of breath, as well as productive cough that has occurred over the past two years for at least three months each year. She is a heavy smoker. | **COPD—chronic bronchitis** Bronchiectasis Lung cancer Tuberculosis CBC | Sputum Gram stain and culture CXR PFTs CT—chest Purified protein derivative (PPD) |

| Presentation | Differential | Workup |
|---|---|---|
| 58 yo M presents with pleuritic chest pain, fever, chills, and cough with purulent yellow sputum. He is a heavy smoker with COPD. | **Pneumonia** <br> Bronchitis <br> Lung abscess <br> Lung cancer <br> Tuberculosis <br> Pericarditis | CBC <br> Sputum Gram stain and culture <br> CXR <br> CT—chest <br> ECG <br> PPD |
| 25 yo F presents with two weeks of a nonproductive cough. Three weeks ago she had a sore throat and a runny nose. | **Atypical pneumonia** <br> Reactive airway disease <br> URI-associated <br> ("postinfectious") <br> Postnasal drip <br> GERD | CBC <br> Induced sputum Gram stain <br> and culture <br> CXR <br> IgM detection for *Mycoplasma pneumoniae* <br> Urine *Legionella* antigen |
| 65 yo M presents with worsening cough over the past six months together with hemoptysis, dyspnea, weakness, and weight loss. He is a heavy smoker. | **Lung cancer** <br> Tuberculosis <br> Lung abscess <br> COPD <br> Vasculitis (i.e., Wegener's) <br> Interstitial lung disease <br> CHF | CBC <br> Sputum Gram stain, culture, <br> and cytology <br> CXR <br> CT—chest <br> PPD <br> Bronchoscopy |
| 55 yo M presents with increased dyspnea and sputum production over the past three days. He has COPD and stopped using his inhalers last week. He also stopped smoking two days ago. | **COPD exacerbation** <br> **(bronchitis)** <br> Lung cancer <br> Pneumonia <br> URI <br> CHF | CBC <br> CXR <br> PFTs <br> Sputum Gram stain and culture <br> CT—chest |
| 34 yo F nurse presents with worsening cough of six weeks' duration together with weight loss, fatigue, night sweats, and fever. She has a history of contact with tuberculosis patients at work. | **Tuberculosis** <br> Pneumonia <br> Lung abscess <br> Vasculitis <br> Lymphoma <br> Metastatic cancer <br> HIV/AIDS | CBC <br> PPD <br> Sputum Gram stain, acid-fast <br> stain, and culture <br> CXR <br> CT—chest <br> Bronchoscopy <br> HIV antibody |

| Presentation | Differential | Workup |
|---|---|---|
| ■ 35 yo M presents with shortness of breath and cough. He has had unprotected sex with multiple sexual partners and was recently exposed to a patient with active tuberculosis. | **Tuberculosis**<br>Pneumonia (including PCP)<br>Bronchitis<br>CHF (cardiomyopathy)<br>Asthma | CBC<br>PPD<br>Sputum Gram stain, acid-fast stain, silver stain, and culture<br>CXR<br>HIV antibody |
| ■ 50 yo M presents with cough that is exacerbated by lying down at night and improved by propping up on three pillows. He also reports exertional dyspnea. | **CHF**<br>Cardiac valvular disease<br>GERD<br>Pulmonary fibrosis<br>COPD<br>Postnasal drip | CBC<br>CXR<br>ECG<br>Echocardiography<br>PFTs<br>BNP |

## ▶ CHEST PAIN

### Key History

Location, quality, severity, radiation, duration, context (exertional, postprandial, positional, cocaine use, trauma), associated symptoms (sweating, nausea, dyspnea, palpitation, sense of doom), exacerbating and alleviating factors (especially medicines); prior history of similar symptoms; known heart or lung disease or history of diagnostic testing; cardiac risk factors (hypertension, hyperlipidemia, smoking, family history of early MI); pulmonary embolism risk factors (history of DVT, coagulopathy, malignancy, recent immobilization).

### Key Physical Exam

Vital signs ± BP in both arms; complete cardiovascular exam (JVD, PMI, chest wall tenderness, heart sounds, pulses, edema); lung and abdominal exams.

| Presentation | Differential | Workup |
|---|---|---|
| ■ 60 yo M presents with sudden onset of substernal heavy chest pain that has lasted for 30 minutes and radiates to the left arm. The pain is accompanied by dyspnea, diaphoresis, and nausea. He has a history of hypertension, hyperlipidemia, and smoking. | **Myocardial infarction (MI)**<br>GERD<br>Angina<br>Costochondritis<br>Aortic dissection<br>Pericarditis<br>Pulmonary embolism<br>Pneumothorax | ECG<br>CPK-MB, troponin<br>CXR<br>CBC, electrolytes<br>Echocardiography<br>Cardiac catheterization |

| Presentation | Differential | Workup |
|---|---|---|
| 20 yo African-American F presents with acute onset of severe chest pain. She has a history of sickle cell disease and multiple previous hospitalizations for pain and anemia management. | **Sickle cell disease—pulmonary infarction**<br>Pneumonia<br>Pulmonary embolism<br>MI<br>Pneumothorax<br>Aortic dissection | CBC, reticulocyte count, LDH, peripheral smear<br>ABG<br>CXR<br>CPK-MB, troponin<br>ECG<br>V/Q scan<br>CT—chest with IV contrast |
| 45 yo F presents with a retrosternal burning sensation that occurs after heavy meals and when lying down. Her symptoms are relieved by antacids. | **GERD**<br>Esophagitis<br>Peptic ulcer disease<br>Esophageal spasm<br>MI<br>Angina | ECG<br>Barium swallow<br>Upper endoscopy<br>Esophageal pH monitoring |
| 55 yo M presents with retrosternal squeezing pain that lasts for two minutes and occurs with exercise. It is relieved by rest and is not related to food intake. | **Angina**<br>GERD<br>Esophageal spasm<br>Esophagitis | ECG<br>CPK-MB, troponin<br>CXR<br>CBC, electrolytes<br>Exercise stress test<br>Upper endoscopy/pH monitor<br>Cardiac catheterization |
| 34 yo F presents with retrosternal stabbing chest pain that improves when she leans forward and worsens with deep inspiration. She had a URI one week ago. | **Pericarditis**<br>Aortic dissection<br>MI<br>Costochondritis<br>GERD<br>Esophageal rupture | ECG<br>CPK-MB, troponin<br>CXR<br>Echocardiography<br>CBC<br>Upper endoscopy |
| 34 yo F presents with stabbing chest pain that worsens with deep inspiration and is relieved by aspirin. She had a URI one week ago. Chest wall tenderness is noted. | **Costochondritis**<br>Pneumonia<br>MI<br>Pulmonary embolism<br>Pericarditis<br>Muscle strain | ECG<br>CPK-MB, troponin<br>CXR<br>CBC |

| Presentation | Differential | Workup |
|---|---|---|
| ▪ 70 yo F presents with acute onset of shortness of breath at rest and pleuritic chest pain. She also presents with tachycardia, hypotension, tachypnea, and mild fever. She is recovering from hip replacement surgery. | **Pulmonary embolism**<br>Pneumonia<br>Costochondritis<br>MI<br>CHF<br>Aortic dissection | ECG<br>CXR<br>ABG<br>CPK-MB, troponin<br>CBC, electrolytes<br>CT—chest with IV contrast<br>Doppler U/S—legs<br>D-dimer |
| ▪ 55 yo M presents with sudden onset of severe chest pain that radiates to the back. He has a history of uncontrolled hypertension. | **Aortic dissection**<br>MI<br>Pericarditis<br>Esophageal rupture<br>Esophageal spasm<br>GERD<br>Pancreatitis | ECG, CPK-MB, troponin<br>CXR<br>CBC, amylase, lipase<br>Transesophageal echocardiography (TEE), MRI/MRA—aorta<br>Aortic angiography<br>Upper endoscopy |

## ▶ PALPITATIONS

### Key History

Gradual vs. acute onset/offset, context (exertion, caffeine, anxiety), associated symptoms (lightheadedness, chest pain, dyspnea); hyperthyroid symptoms; history of bleeding or anemia; history of heart disease.

### Key Physical Exam

Vital signs; endocrine/thyroid exam, including exophthalmos, lid retraction, lid lag, gland size, bruit, and tremor; complete cardiovascular exam.

| Presentation | Differential | Workup |
|---|---|---|
| ▪ 70 yo diabetic M presents with episodes of palpitations and diaphoresis. He is on insulin. | **Hypoglycemia**<br>Cardiac arrhythmias<br>Angina<br>Hyperthyroidism<br>Hyperventilation episodes<br>Panic attacks<br>Pheochromocytoma<br>Carcinoid | Glucose<br>CBC, electrolytes<br>TSH<br>BUN/Cr<br>ECG<br>Holter monitor |

## Key History

Amount, duration, ± intentional; diet history, body image, anxiety or depression; other constitutional symptoms; palpitation, tremor, diarrhea, family history of thyroid disease; HIV risk factors; alcohol and drug use; medications; history of cancer.

## Key Physical Exam

Vital signs; complete physical.

| Presentation | Differential | Workup |
|---|---|---|
| ▪ 42 yo F presents with a 7-kg weight loss over the past two months. She has a fine tremor, and her pulse is 112. | **Hyperthyroidism**<br>Cancer<br>HIV infection<br>Dieting/diet drugs<br>Anorexia nervosa<br>Malabsorption | TSH, $FT_4$<br>CBC, electrolytes<br>HIV antibody<br>Urine toxicology |

## Key History

Amount, duration, timing (relation to medication changes, smoking cessation, depression); diet history; hypothyroid symptoms (fatigue, constipation, skin/hair/nail changes); menstrual irregularity; past medical history; alcohol and drug use.

## Key Physical Exam

Vital signs; complete exam, including signs of Cushing's syndrome (hypertension, central obesity, moon face, buffalo hump, supraclavicular fat pads, purple abdominal striae).

| Presentation | Differential | Workup |
|---|---|---|
| ▪ 44 yo F presents with a weight gain of > 11 kg over the past two months. She quit smoking three months ago and is on amitriptyline for depression. She also reports cold intolerance and constipation. | **Smoking cessation**<br>Drug side effect<br>Hypothyroidism<br>Cushing's syndrome<br>Polycystic ovary syndrome<br>Diabetes mellitus<br>Depression | CBC, electrolytes, glucose<br>TSH<br>24-hour urine free cortisol<br>Dexamethasone suppression test |

## Key History

Solids vs. both solids and liquids, ± progressive, constitutional symptoms (especially weight loss), drooling, regurgitation, odynophagia, GERD symptoms; medications; HIV risk factors, history of smoking, history of Raynaud's phenomenon.

## Key Physical Exam

Vital signs; head and neck exam; heart, lung, and abdominal exams; skin exam (for signs of scleroderma/CREST).

| Presentation | Differential | Workup |
| --- | --- | --- |
| 75 yo M presents with dysphagia that started with solids and progressed to liquids. He is an alcoholic and a heavy smoker. He has had an unintentional weight loss of 7 kg over the past four months. | **Esophageal cancer**<br>Achalasia<br>Esophagitis<br>Systemic sclerosis<br>Esophageal stricture<br>Amyotrophic lateral sclerosis | CBC<br>CXR<br>Endoscopy with biopsy<br>Barium swallow<br>CT—chest |
| 45 yo F presents with dysphagia for two weeks together with fatigue and a craving for ice and clay. | **Plummer-Vinson syndrome**<br>Esophageal cancer<br>Esophagitis<br>Achalasia<br>Systemic sclerosis<br>Mitral valve stenosis | CBC<br>Serum iron, ferritin, TIBC<br>Barium swallow<br>Endoscopy |
| 48 yo F presents with dysphagia for both solid and liquid foods that has slowly progressed in severity over the past year. It is associated with regurgitation of undigested food, especially at night. | **Achalasia**<br>Plummer-Vinson syndrome<br>Esophageal cancer<br>Esophagitis<br>Systemic sclerosis<br>Mitral valve stenosis<br>Esophageal stricture<br>Zenker's diverticulum | CXR<br>Endoscopy<br>Barium swallow<br>Esophageal manometry |
| 38 yo M presents with dysphagia and pain on swallowing solids more than liquids. Exam reveals oral thrush. | **Esophagitis** (CMV, HSV, pill-induced)<br>Systemic sclerosis<br>GERD<br>Esophageal stricture<br>Zenker's diverticulum | CBC<br>Endoscopy<br>Barium swallow<br>HIV antibody<br>CD4 count |

### Key History

Acuity of onset, ± abdominal pain, relation to meals, sick contacts, possible food poisoning, possible pregnancy; neurologic symptoms (headache, stiff neck, vertigo, focal numbness or weakness), other associated symptoms (GI, chest pain), exacerbating and alleviating factors; medications.

### Key Physical Exam

Vital signs; ENT; consider funduscopic exam (increased intracranial pressure); complete abdominal exam; consider heart, lung, and rectal exams.

| Presentation | Differential | Workup |
|---|---|---|
| ▪ 20 yo F presents with nausea, vomiting (especially in the morning), fatigue, and polyuria. Her last menstrual period was six weeks ago, and her breasts are full and tender. She is sexually active with her boyfriend, and they use condoms for contraception. | **Pregnancy**<br>Gastritis<br>Hypercalcemia<br>Diabetes mellitus<br>UTI<br>Depression | Urine hCG<br>Pelvic exam<br>U/S—pelvis<br>CBC, electrolytes, calcium, glucose<br>UA, urine culture<br>Baseline Pap smear, cervical cultures, rubella antibodies, HIV antibody, hepatitis B surface antigen, and RPR/VDRL |

### Key History

Location, quality, intensity, duration, radiation, timing (relation to meals), associated symptoms (constitutional, GI, cardiac, pulmonary, renal, pelvic, other), exacerbating and alleviating factors; prior history of similar symptoms; history of abdominal surgeries, gallstones, renal stones, atherosclerotic vascular disease; medications; alcohol and drug use; domestic violence.

### Key Physical Exam

Vital signs; heart and lung exams; abdominal exam, including guarding, rebound, Murphy's sign, and CVA palpation; rectal exam; pelvic exam (women).

| Presentation | Differential | Workup |
|---|---|---|
| ▪ 45 yo M presents with sudden onset of colicky right-sided flank pain that radiates to the testicles, accompanied by nausea, vomiting, hematuria, and CVA tenderness. | **Nephrolithiasis**<br>Renal cell carcinoma<br>Pyelonephritis<br>GI etiology (e.g., appendicitis) | Rectal exam<br>UA<br>Urine culture and sensitivity<br>BUN/Cr<br>CT—abdomen<br>U/S—renal<br>IVP |
| ▪ 60 yo M presents with dull epigastric pain that radiates to the back, together with weight loss, dark urine, and clay-colored stool. He is a heavy drinker and smoker. | **Pancreatic cancer**<br>Acute viral hepatitis<br>Chronic pancreatitis<br>Cholecystitis/choledocholithiasis<br>Abdominal aortic aneurysm<br>Peptic ulcer disease | Rectal exam<br>CBC, electrolytes<br>Amylase and lipase<br>AST/ALT/bilirubin/alkaline phosphatase<br>U/S—abdomen<br>CT—abdomen |
| ▪ 56 yo M presents with severe midepigastric abdominal pain that radiates to the back and improves when he leans forward. He also reports anorexia, nausea, and vomiting. He is an alcoholic and has spent the past three days binge drinking. | **Acute pancreatitis**<br>Peptic ulcer disease<br>Cholecystitis/choledocholithiasis<br>Gastritis<br>Abdominal aortic aneurysm<br>Mesenteric ischemia<br>Alcoholic hepatitis<br>Mallory-Weiss tear | Rectal exam<br>CBC, electrolytes, BUN/Cr, amylase, lipase, AST/ALT/ bilirubin/alkaline phosphatase<br>U/S—abdomen<br>CT—abdomen<br>Upper endoscopy<br>ECG |
| ▪ 41 yo obese F presents with RUQ abdominal pain that radiates to the right scapula and is associated with nausea, vomiting, and a fever of 101.5°F. The pain started after she had eaten fatty food. She has had similar but less intense episodes that lasted a few hours. Exam reveals positive Murphy's sign. | **Acute cholecystitis**<br>Hepatitis<br>Choledocholithiasis<br>Ascending cholangitis<br>Peptic ulcer disease<br>Fitz-Hugh–Curtis syndrome | Rectal exam<br>CBC<br>AST/ALT/bilirubin/alkaline phosphatase<br>U/S—abdomen<br>HIDA scan |
| ▪ 43 yo obese F presents with RUQ abdominal pain, fever, and jaundice. She was diagnosed with asymptomatic gallstones one year ago. | **Ascending cholangitis**<br>Acute cholecystitis<br>Hepatitis<br>Choledocholithiasis<br>Sclerosing cholangitis<br>Fitz-Hugh–Curtis syndrome | Rectal exam<br>CBC<br>AST/ALT/bilirubin/alkaline phosphatase<br>Viral hepatitis serologies<br>U/S—abdomen<br>MRCP<br>ERCP |

| Presentation | Differential | Workup |
|---|---|---|
| ■ 25 yo M presents with RUQ pain, fever, anorexia, nausea, and vomiting. He has dark urine and clay-colored stool. | **Acute hepatitis** Acute cholecystitis Ascending cholangitis Choledocholithiasis Pancreatitis Acute glomerulonephritis | Rectal exam CBC, amylase, lipase AST/ALT/bilirubin/alkaline phosphatase UA Viral hepatitis serologies U/S—abdomen |
| ■ 35 yo M presents with burning epigastric pain that starts 2–3 hours after meals. The pain is relieved by food and antacids. | **Peptic ulcer disease** Gastritis GERD Cholecystitis Chronic pancreatitis Mesenteric ischemia | Rectal exam Amylase, lipase, lactate AST/ALT/bilirubin/alkaline phosphatase Endoscopy (including *H. pylori* testing) Upper GI series |
| ■ 37 yo M presents with severe epigastric pain, nausea, vomiting, and mild fever. He appears toxic. He has a history of intermittent epigastric pain that is relieved by food and antacids. He also smokes heavily and takes aspirin on a regular basis. | **Peptic ulcer perforation** Acute pancreatitis Hepatitis Cholecystitis Choledocholithiasis Mesenteric ischemia | Rectal exam CBC, electrolytes, amylase, lipase, lactate AST/ALT/bilirubin/alkaline phosphatase AXR Upright CXR Endoscopy (including *H. pylori* testing) |
| ■ 18 yo M boxer presents with severe LUQ abdominal pain that radiates to the left scapula. He had infectious mononucleosis three weeks ago. | **Splenic rupture** Kidney stone Rib fracture Pneumonia Perforated peptic ulcer Splenic infarct | Rectal exam CBC, electrolytes CXR CT—abdomen U/S—abdomen |
| ■ 40 yo M presents with crampy abdominal pain, vomiting, abdominal distention, and inability to pass flatus or stool. He has a history of multiple abdominal surgeries. | **Intestinal obstruction** Small bowel or colon cancer Volvulus of the bowel Gastroenteritis Food poisoning Ileus | Rectal exam CBC, electrolytes AXR CT—abdomen/pelvis CXR |

MINICASES

| Presentation | Differential | Workup |
|---|---|---|
| ▪ 70 yo F presents with acute onset of severe, crampy abdominal pain. She recently vomited and had a massive dark bowel movement. She has a history of CHF and atrial fibrillation, for which she has received digitalis. Her pain is out of proportion to the exam. | **Mesenteric ischemia/infarction** <br> Diverticulitis <br> Peptic ulcer disease <br> Gastroenteritis <br> Acute pancreatitis <br> Cholecystitis/choledocholithiasis <br> MI | Rectal exam <br> CBC, amylase, lipase, lactate <br> ECG, CPK-MB, troponin <br> AXR <br> CT—abdomen <br> Mesenteric angiography <br> Barium enema |
| ▪ 21 yo F presents with acute onset of severe RLQ pain, nausea, and vomiting. She has no fever, urinary symptoms, or vaginal bleeding and has never taken OCPs. Her last menstrual period was regular, and she has no history of STDs. | **Ovarian torsion** <br> Appendicitis <br> Nephrolithiasis <br> Ectopic pregnancy <br> Ruptured ovarian cyst <br> PID <br> Bowel infarction or perforation | Pelvic exam <br> Rectal exam <br> Urine hCG <br> UA <br> CBC <br> Doppler U/S—pelvis <br> CT—abdomen <br> Laparoscopy |
| ▪ 68 yo M presents with lower LLQ abdominal pain, fever, and chills for the past three days. He also reports recent onset of alternating diarrhea and constipation. He consumes a low-fiber, high-fat diet. | **Diverticulitis** <br> Crohn's disease <br> Ulcerative colitis <br> Gastroenteritis <br> Abscess | Rectal exam <br> CBC, electrolytes <br> CXR <br> AXR <br> CT—abdomen |
| ▪ 20 yo M presents with severe RLQ abdominal pain, nausea, and vomiting. His discomfort started yesterday as a vague pain around the umbilicus. As the pain worsened, it became sharp and migrated to the RLQ. McBurney's and psoas signs are positive. | **Acute appendicitis** <br> Gastroenteritis <br> Diverticulitis <br> Crohn's disease <br> Nephrolithiasis <br> Volvulus or other intestinal obstruction/perforation | Rectal exam <br> CBC, electrolytes <br> AXR <br> CT—abdomen <br> U/S—abdomen |
| ▪ 30 yo F presents with periumbilical pain for six months. The pain never awakens her from sleep. It is relieved by defecation and worsens when she is upset. She has alternating constipation and diarrhea but no nausea, vomiting, weight loss, or anorexia. | **Irritable bowel syndrome** <br> Crohn's disease <br> Celiac disease <br> Chronic pancreatitis <br> GI parasitic infection (amebiasis, giardiasis) <br> Endometriosis | Rectal exam, stool for occult blood <br> Pelvic exam <br> Urine hCG <br> CBC <br> Electrolytes <br> CT—abdomen/pelvis <br> Stool for ova and parasitology, *Entamoeba histolytica* antigen |

| Presentation | Differential | Workup |
|---|---|---|
| 24 yo F presents with bilateral lower abdominal pain that started with the first day of her menstrual period. The pain is associated with fever and a thick, greenish-yellow vaginal discharge. She has had unprotected sex with multiple sexual partners. | **PID** <br> Endometriosis <br> Dysmenorrhea <br> Vaginitis <br> Cystitis <br> Spontaneous abortion <br> Pyelonephritis | Pelvic exam <br> Rectal exam <br> Urine hCG <br> Cervical cultures <br> CBC/ESR <br> UA, urine culture <br> U/S—pelvis |

► CONSTIPATION/DIARRHEA

### Key History

Frequency and volume of stools, duration of change in bowel habits, associated symptoms (constitutional, abdominal pain, bloating, sense of incomplete evacuation, melena or hematochezia); thyroid disease symptoms; diet (especially fiber and fluid intake); medications (including recent antibiotics); sick contacts, travel, camping, HIV risk factors; history of abdominal surgeries, diabetes, pancreatitis; alcohol and drug use; family history of colon cancer.

### Key Physical Exam

Vital signs; relevant thyroid/endocrine exam; abdominal and rectal exams; ± female pelvic exam.

| Presentation | Differential | Workup |
|---|---|---|
| 67 yo M presents with alternating diarrhea and constipation, decreased stool caliber, and blood in the stool for the past eight months. He also reports unintentional weight loss. He is on a low-fiber diet and has a family history of colon cancer. | **Colorectal cancer** <br> Irritable bowel syndrome <br> Diverticulosis <br> GI parasitic infection (ascariasis, giardiasis) <br> Inflammatory bowel disease <br> Angiodysplasia | Rectal exam <br> CBC <br> AST/ALT/bilirubin/alkaline phosphatase <br> CEA <br> Colonoscopy <br> Barium enema <br> CT—abdomen/pelvis |
| 28 yo M presents with constipation (very hard stool) for the last three weeks. Since his mother died two months ago, he and his father have eaten only junk food. | **Low-fiber diet** <br> Irritable bowel syndrome <br> Substance abuse (e.g., heroin) <br> Depression <br> Hypothyroidism | Rectal exam <br> TSH <br> Electrolytes <br> Urine toxicology |

| Presentation | Differential | Workup |
|---|---|---|
| ▪ 30 yo F presents with alternating constipation and diarrhea and abdominal pain that is relieved by defecation. She has no nausea, vomiting, weight loss, or blood in her stool. | **Irritable bowel syndrome** <br> Inflammatory bowel disease <br> Celiac disease <br> Chronic pancreatitis <br> GI parasitic infection (ascariasis, giardiasis) <br> Lactose intolerance | Rectal exam, stool for occult blood <br> CBC <br> Electrolytes <br> Stool for ova and parasitology <br> AXR <br> CT—abdomen/pelvis |
| ▪ 33 yo M presents with watery diarrhea, vomiting, and diffuse abdominal pain that began yesterday. He also reports feeling hot. Several of his coworkers are also ill. | **Infectious diarrhea (gastroenteritis)**—bacterial, viral, parasitic, protozoal <br> Food poisoning <br> Inflammatory bowel disease | Rectal exam, stool for occult blood <br> Stool leukocytes and culture <br> CBC <br> Electrolytes <br> CT—abdomen/pelvis |
| ▪ 40 yo F presents with watery diarrhea and abdominal cramps. Last week she was on antibiotics for a UTI. | **Pseudomembranous (*Clostridium difficile*) colitis** <br> Gastroenteritis <br> Cryptosporidiosis <br> Food poisoning <br> Inflammatory bowel disease | Rectal exam <br> Stool leukocytes, culture, occult blood <br> *C. difficile* toxin in stool <br> Electrolytes |
| ▪ 25 yo M presents with watery diarrhea and abdominal cramps. He was recently in Mexico. | **Traveler's diarrhea** <br> Giardiasis <br> Amebiasis <br> Food poisoning <br> Hepatitis A | Rectal exam <br> Stool leukocytes, culture, *Giardia* antigen, *Entamoeba histolytica* antigen <br> Electrolytes <br> AST/ALT/bilirubin/alkaline phosphatase <br> Viral hepatitis serology |
| ▪ 30 yo F presents with watery diarrhea and abdominal cramping and bloating. Her symptoms are aggravated by milk ingestion and are relieved by fasting. | **Lactose intolerance** <br> Gastroenteritis <br> Inflammatory bowel disease <br> Irritable bowel syndrome <br> Hyperthyroidism | Rectal exam <br> Stool exam <br> Hydrogen breath test <br> TSH |
| ▪ 33 yo M presents with watery diarrhea, diffuse abdominal pain, and weight loss over the past three weeks. He has not responded to antibiotics. | **Crohn's disease** <br> Gastroenteritis <br> Ulcerative colitis <br> Celiac disease <br> Pseudomembranous colitis <br> Hyperthyroidism <br> Small bowel lymphoma | Rectal exam <br> Stool exam and culture <br> CBC, electrolytes <br> TSH <br> CT—abdomen <br> Colonoscopy <br> Small bowel series |

MINICASES

### Key History

Amount, duration, context (after severe vomiting, alcohol ingestion, nosebleed), associated symptoms (constitutional, nausea, abdominal pain, dyspepsia); medications (especially warfarin, NSAIDs); history of peptic ulcer disease, liver disease, abdominal aortic aneurysm repair, easy bleeding.

### Key Physical Exam

Vital signs, including orthostatics; ENT, heart, lung, abdominal, and rectal exams.

| Presentation | Differential | Workup |
|---|---|---|
| 45 yo F presents with coffee-ground emesis for the last three days. Her stool is dark and tarry. She has a history of intermittent epigastric pain that is relieved by food and antacids. | **Bleeding peptic ulcer**<br>Gastritis<br>Gastric cancer<br>Esophageal varices | Rectal exam<br>CBC, electrolytes<br>AST/ALT/bilirubin/alkaline phosphatase<br>Endoscopy (including *H. pylori* testing if ulcer is confirmed) |
| 40 yo F presents with epigastric pain and coffee-ground emesis. She has a history of rheumatoid arthritis that has been treated with aspirin. She is an alcoholic. | **Gastritis**<br>Bleeding peptic ulcer<br>Gastric cancer<br>Esophageal varices<br>Mallory-Weiss tear | Rectal exam<br>CBC, electrolytes<br>AST/ALT/bilirubin/alkaline phosphatase<br>Barium swallow<br>Endoscopy |

### Key History

Melena vs. bright blood; amount, duration, associated symptoms (constitutional, abdominal or rectal pain, tenesmus, constipation/diarrhea); trauma; prior history of similar symptoms; prior colonoscopy; medications (especially warfarin); history of easy bleeding or atherosclerotic vascular disease.

### Key Physical Exam

Vital signs ± orthostatics; abdominal and rectal exams.

| Presentation | Differential | Workup |
|---|---|---|
| 67 yo M presents with blood in his stool, weight loss, and constipation. He has a family history of colon cancer. | **Colorectal cancer**<br>Anal fissure<br>Hemorrhoids<br>Diverticulosis<br>Ischemic bowel disease<br>Angiodysplasia<br>Upper GI bleeding<br>Inflammatory bowel disease | Rectal exam<br>CBC, PT/PTT<br>AST/ALT/bilirubin/alkaline<br>   phosphatase<br>CEA<br>Colonoscopy<br>CT—abdomen/pelvis<br>Barium enema |
| 33 yo F presents with rectal bleeding and diarrhea for the past week. She has had lower abdominal pain and tenesmus for several months. | **Ulcerative colitis**<br>Crohn's disease<br>Proctitis<br>Anal fissure<br>Hemorrhoids<br>Diverticulosis<br>Dysentery | Rectal exam<br>CBC, PT/PTT<br>AXR<br>Colonoscopy<br>CT—abdomen/pelvis<br>Barium enema |
| 58 yo M presents with bright red blood per rectum and chronic constipation. He consumes a low-fiber diet. | **Diverticulosis**<br>Anal fissure<br>Hemorrhoids<br>Angiodysplasia<br>Colorectal cancer | Rectal exam<br>CBC, PT/PTT<br>Electrolytes<br>Colonoscopy<br>CT—abdomen/pelvis |

▶ **HEMATURIA**

## Key History

Amount, duration, ± clots, associated symptoms (constitutional, renal colic, dysuria, irritative voiding symptoms); medications; history of vigorous exercise, trauma, smoking, stones, cancer, or easy bleeding.

## Key Physical Exam

Vital signs; lymph nodes; abdominal exam; genitourinary and rectal exams; extremities.

| Presentation | Differential | Workup |
|---|---|---|
| ■ 65 yo M presents with painless hematuria. He is a heavy smoker and works as a painter. | **Bladder cancer**<br>Renal cell carcinoma<br>Nephrolithiasis<br>Acute glomerulonephritis<br>Prostate cancer<br>Coagulation disorder (i.e., factor VIII antibodies)<br>Polycystic kidney disease | Genitourinary exam<br>UA, urine cytology<br>BUN/Cr, PSA, CBC, PT/PTT<br>Cystoscopy<br>U/S—renal/bladder<br>CT—abdomen/pelvis<br>IVP |
| ■ 35 yo M presents with painless hematuria. He has a family history of kidney problems. | **Polycystic kidney disease**<br>Nephrolithiasis<br>Acute glomerulonephritis (e.g., IgA nephropathy)<br>UTI<br>Coagulation disorder<br>Bladder cancer | Genitourinary exam<br>UA<br>BUN/Cr, PSA, CBC, PT/PTT<br>U/S—renal<br>CT—abdomen/pelvis<br>IVP |
| ■ 55 yo M presents with flank pain and blood in his urine without dysuria. He has experienced weight loss and fever over the past two months. | **Renal cell carcinoma**<br>Bladder cancer<br>Nephrolithiasis<br>Acute glomerulonephritis<br>Pyelonephritis<br>Prostate cancer | Genitourinary, rectal exam<br>UA, urine cytology, BUN/Cr, PSA, CBC, PT/PTT<br>U/S—renal<br>CT—abdomen/pelvis<br>IVP |

► OTHER URINARY SYMPTOMS

### Key History

Duration, obstructive symptoms (hesitancy, diminished stream, sense of incomplete bladder emptying, straining, postvoid dribbling), irritative symptoms (urgency, frequency, nocturia), constitutional symptoms; bone pain; medications; history of UTIs, urethral stricture, or urinary tract instrumentation; stones, diabetes, alcoholism.

### Key Physical Exam

Vital signs; abdominal exam (including suprapubic percussion to assess for a distended bladder); genital and rectal exams; focused neurologic exam.

MINICASES

| Presentation | Differential | Workup |
|---|---|---|
| 60 yo M presents with nocturia, urgency, weak stream, and terminal dribbling. He denies any weight loss, fatigue, or bone pain. He has had two episodes of urinary retention that required catheterization. | **Benign prostatic hypertrophy (BPH)**<br>Prostate cancer<br>UTI<br>Bladder stones | Rectal exam<br>UA<br>CBC, BUN/Cr, PSA<br>U/S—prostate (transrectal) |
| 71 yo M presents with nocturia, urgency, weak stream, terminal dribbling, hematuria, and lower back pain over the past four months. He has also experienced weight loss and fatigue. | **Prostate cancer**<br>BPH<br>Renal cell carcinoma<br>UTI<br>Bladder stones | Rectal exam<br>UA<br>CBC, BUN/Cr, PSA<br>U/S—prostate (transrectal)<br>CT—pelvis<br>IVP |
| 18 yo M presents with a burning sensation during urination and urethral discharge. He recently had unprotected sex with a new partner. | **Urethritis**<br>Cystitis<br>Prostatitis | Genital ± rectal exam<br>UA<br>Urine culture<br>Gram stain and culture of urethral discharge<br>Chlamydia and gonorrhea PCR |
| 45 yo diabetic F presents with dysuria, urinary frequency, fever, chills, and nausea over the past three days. There is left CVA tenderness on exam. | **Acute pyelonephritis**<br>Nephrolithiasis<br>Renal cell carcinoma<br>Lower UTI (cystitis, urethritis) | UA<br>Urine culture and sensitivity<br>CBC, BUN/Cr<br>U/S—renal<br>CT—abdomen |

► **ERECTILE DYSFUNCTION (ED)**

## Key History

Duration, severity, ± nocturnal erections, libido, stress or depression, trauma, associated incontinence; medications (and recent changes); past medical history (hypertension, diabetes, high cholesterol, known atherosclerotic vascular disease, prior prostate surgery); smoking, alcohol and drug use.

## Key Physical Exam

Vital signs; cardiovascular exam; genital and rectal exams.

| Presentation | Differential | Workup |
|---|---|---|
| 47 yo M presents with impotence that started three months ago. He has hypertension and was started on atenolol four months ago. He also has diabetes and is on insulin. | **Drug-related ED**<br>ED caused by hypertension<br>ED caused by diabetes mellitus<br>Psychogenic ED<br>Peyronie's disease | Genital exam<br>Rectal exam<br>Glucose<br>CBC |

**Key History**

Primary vs. secondary, duration, possible pregnancy, associated symptoms (headache, decreased peripheral vision, galactorrhea, hirsutism, virilization, hot flushes, vaginal dryness, symptoms of thyroid disease); history of anorexia nervosa, excessive dieting, vigorous exercise, pregnancies, D&Cs, uterine infections; drug use; medications.

**Key Physical Exam**

Vital signs; breast exam; complete pelvic exam.

| Presentation | Differential | Workup |
|---|---|---|
| ■ 40 yo F presents with amenorrhea, morning nausea and vomiting, fatigue, and polyuria. Her last menstrual period was six weeks ago, and her breasts are full and tender. She uses the rhythm method for contraception. | **Pregnancy**<br>Anovulatory cycle<br>Hyperprolactinemia<br>UTI<br>Thyroid disease | Pelvic exam<br>Urine hCG<br>U/S—pelvis<br>CBC, electrolytes<br>UA, urine culture<br>Prolactin, TSH<br>Baseline Pap smear, cervical cultures, rubella antibody, HIV antibody, hepatitis B surface antigen, and RPR/VDRL |
| ■ 23 yo obese F presents with amenorrhea for six months, facial hair, and infertility for the past three years. | **Polycystic ovary syndrome**<br>Thyroid disease<br>Hyperprolactinemia<br>Pregnancy<br>Ovarian or adrenal malignancy<br>Premature ovarian failure | Pelvic exam<br>Urine hCG<br>U/S—pelvis<br>LH/FSH, TSH, prolactin<br>Testosterone, DHEAS |
| ■ 35 yo F presents with amenorrhea, galactorrhea, visual field defects, and headaches for the past six months. | **Amenorrhea secondary to prolactinoma**<br>Pregnancy<br>Thyroid disease<br>Premature ovarian failure<br>Pituitary tumor | Pelvic and breast exam<br>Urine hCG<br>Prolactin<br>LH/FSH, TSH<br>MRI—brain |
| ■ 48 yo F presents with amenorrhea for the past six months accompanied by hot flushes, night sweats, emotional lability, and dyspareunia. | **Menopause**<br>Pregnancy<br>Pituitary tumor<br>Thyroid disease | Pelvic exam<br>Urine hCG<br>LH/FSH, TSH, prolactin, testosterone, DHEAS<br>CBC<br>MRI—brain |

MINICASES

| Presentation | Differential | Workup |
|---|---|---|
| 35 yo F presents with amenorrhea, cold intolerance, coarse hair, weight loss, and fatigue. She has a history of abruptio placentae followed by hypovolemic shock and failure of lactation two years ago. | **Sheehan's syndrome**<br>Premature ovarian failure<br>Pituitary tumor<br>Thyroid disease<br>Asherman's syndrome | Pelvic exam<br>Urine hCG<br>CBC<br>LH/FSH, prolactin<br>TSH, $FT_4$<br>ACTH<br>MRI—brain<br>Hysteroscopy |
| 18 yo F presents with amenorrhea for the past four months. She has lost 95 pounds and has a history of vigorous exercise and cold intolerance. | **Anorexia nervosa** | CBC<br>TSH<br>$FT_4$<br>ACTH<br>FSH<br>LH |
| 29 yo F presents with amenorrhea for the past six months. She has a history of occasional palpitation and dizziness. She lost her fiancé in a car accident. | **Anxiety-induced amenorrhea** | CBC<br>TSH<br>$FT_4$<br>ACTH<br>Urine cortisol level<br>Progesterone challenge test |

▶ **VAGINAL BLEEDING**

## Key History

Pre- vs. postmenopausal, duration, amount; menstrual history and relation to last menstrual period; associated discharge, pelvic or abdominal pain, or urinary symptoms; trauma; medications (especially warfarin, contraceptives); history of easy bleeding or bruising; history of abnormal Pap smears.

## Key Physical Exam

Vital signs; abdominal exam; complete pelvic exam.

| Presentation | Differential | Workup |
|---|---|---|
| 17 yo F presents with prolonged, excessive menstrual bleeding occurring irregularly over the past six months. | **Dysfunctional uterine bleeding**<br>Coagulation disorders (e.g., von Willebrand's disease, hemophilia)<br>Cervical cancer<br>Molar pregnancy<br>Hypothyroidism<br>Diabetes mellitus | Pelvic exam<br>Urine hCG<br>Cervical cultures, Pap smear<br>CBC, ESR, glucose<br>PT/PTT<br>Prolactin, FSH/LH<br>TSH<br>U/S—pelvis |

| Presentation | Differential | Workup |
|---|---|---|
| 61 yo obese F presents with profuse vaginal bleeding over the past month. Her last menstrual period was 10 years ago. She has a history of hypertension and diabetes mellitus. She is nulliparous. | **Endometrial cancer** <br> Cervical cancer <br> Atrophic endometrium <br> Endometrial hyperplasia <br> Endometrial polyps <br> Atrophic vaginitis | Pelvic exam <br> Pap smear <br> Endometrial biopsy <br> U/S—pelvis <br> Endometrial curettage <br> Colposcopy <br> Hysteroscopy |
| 45 yo G5P5 F presents with postcoital bleeding. She is a cigarette smoker and takes OCPs. | **Cervical cancer** <br> Cervical polyp <br> Cervicitis <br> Trauma (e.g., cervical laceration) | Pelvic exam <br> Pap smear <br> Colposcopy and biopsy |
| 28 yo F who is eight weeks pregnant presents with lower abdominal pain and vaginal bleeding. | **Spontaneous abortion** <br> Ectopic pregnancy <br> Molar pregnancy | Pelvic exam <br> Urine hCG <br> U/S—pelvis <br> CBC, PT/PTT <br> Quantitive serum hCG |
| 32 yo F presents with sudden onset of left lower abdominal pain that radiates to the scapula and back and is associated with vaginal bleeding. Her last menstrual period was five weeks ago. She has a history of PID and unprotected intercourse. | **Ectopic pregnancy** <br> Ruptured ovarian cyst <br> Ovarian torsion <br> PID | Pelvic exam <br> Urine hCG <br> Cervical cultures <br> U/S—pelvis <br> Quantitative serum hCG |

► **VAGINAL DISCHARGE**

## Key History

Amount, color, consistency, odor, duration; associated vaginal burning, pain, or pruritus; recent sexual activity; onset of last menstrual period; use of contraceptives, tampons, and douches; history of similar symptoms; history of STD.

## Key Physical Exam

Vital signs; abdominal exam; complete pelvic exam.

| Presentation | Differential | Workup |
|---|---|---|
| 28 yo F presents with a thin, grayish-white, foul-smelling vaginal discharge. | **Bacterial vaginosis**<br>Vaginitis—candidal<br>Vaginitis—trichomonal<br>Cervicitis (chlamydia, gonorrhea) | Pelvic exam<br>Wet mount<br>Cervical cultures<br>KOH prep ("whiff test")<br>pH of vaginal fluid |
| 30 yo F presents with a thick, white, cottage cheese–like, odorless vaginal discharge and vaginal itching. | **Vaginitis—candidal**<br>Bacterial vaginosis<br>Vaginitis—trichomonal | Pelvic exam<br>KOH prep ("whiff test")<br>Wet mount<br>Cervical cultures<br>pH of vaginal fluid |
| 35 yo F presents with a malodorous, profuse, frothy, greenish vaginal discharge with intense vaginal itching and discomfort. | **Vaginitis—trichomonal**<br>Vaginitis—candidal<br>Bacterial vaginosis<br>Cervicitis (chlamydia, gonorrhea) | Pelvic exam<br>Wet mount<br>Cervical cultures<br>pH of the vaginal fluid<br>KOH prep ("whiff test") |

▶ **DYSPAREUNIA**

## Key History

Duration, timing, associated symptoms (vaginal discharge, rash, painful menses, GI symptoms, hot flushes), adequacy of lubrication; libido; sexual history; history of sexual trauma or domestic violence; history of endometriosis, PID, or prior abdominal/pelvic surgeries.

## Key Physical Exam

Vital signs; abdominal exam; complete pelvic exam.

| Presentation | Differential | Workup |
|---|---|---|
| 54 yo F c/o painful intercourse. Her last menstrual period was nine months ago. She has hot flushes. | **Atrophic vaginitis**<br>Endometriosis<br>Cervicitis<br>Depression<br>Domestic abuse | Pelvic exam<br>Wet mount, KOH prep, cervical cultures<br>U/S—pelvis |

| Presentation | Differential | Workup |
|---|---|---|
| ■ 37 yo F presents with dyspareunia, inability to conceive, and dysmenorrhea. | **Endometriosis**<br>Cervicitis<br>Vaginismus<br>Vulvodynia<br>PID<br>Depression<br>Domestic violence | Pelvic exam<br>Wet mount, KOH prep, cervical cultures<br>U/S—pelvis<br>Laparoscopy |

► **ABUSE**

## Key History

Establish confidentiality; directly question about physical, sexual, or emotional abuse and about fear, safety, backup plan; history of frequent accidents/injuries, mental illness, drug use; firearms in the home.

## Key Physical Exam

Vital signs; complete exam ± pelvic.

| Presentation | Differential | Workup |
|---|---|---|
| ■ 28 yo F c/o multiple facial and bodily injuries. She claims that she fell on the stairs. She was hospitalized for some physical injuries seven months ago. She presents with her husband. | **Domestic violence**<br>Osteogenesis imperfecta<br>Substance abuse<br>Consensual violent sexual behavior | XR—skeletal survey<br>CT—maxillofacial<br>Urine toxicology<br>CBC |
| ■ 30 yo F presents with multiple facial and physical injuries. She was attacked and raped by two men. | **Rape** | Pelvic exam<br>Urine hCG<br>Wet mount, KOH prep, cervical cultures<br>XR—skeletal survey<br>CBC<br>HIV antibody<br>Viral hepatitis serologies |

## Key History

Location, quality, intensity, duration, pattern (small vs. large joints, number involved; swelling, redness, warmth), associated symptoms (constitutional, red eye, oral or genital ulceration, diarrhea, dysuria, rash, focal numbness/weakness), exacerbating and alleviating factors; trauma (including vigorous exercise); medications; DVT risk factors; alcohol and drug use; family history of rheumatic disease.

## Key Physical Exam

Vital signs; HEENT and musculoskeletal exams; relevant neurovascular exam.

| Presentation | Differential | Workup |
|---|---|---|
| 30 yo F presents with wrist pain and a black eye after tripping, falling, and hitting her head on the edge of a table. She looks anxious and gives an inconsistent story. | **Domestic violence** Factitious disorder Substance abuse | XR—wrist CT—head Urine toxicology |
| 30 yo F secretary presents with wrist pain and a sensation of numbness and burning in her palm and the first, second, and third fingers of her right hand. The pain worsens at night and is relieved by loose shaking of the hand. There is sensory loss in the same fingers. Exam reveals positive Tinel's sign. | **Carpal tunnel syndrome** Median nerve compression in forearm or arm | Nerve conduction study XR—wrist MRI—wrist |
| 28 yo F presents with pain in the interphalangeal joints of her hands together with hair loss and a butterfly rash on the face. | **Systemic lupus erythematosus (SLE)** Rheumatoid arthritis Psoriatic arthritis Parvovirus B19 infection | ANA, anti-dsDNA, ESR, C3, C4, rheumatoid factor (RF), CBC XR—hands UA |
| 28 yo F presents with pain in the metacarpophalangeal joints of both hands. Her left knee is also painful and red. She has morning joint stiffness that lasts for an hour. Her mother had rheumatoid arthritis. | **Rheumatoid arthritis** SLE Disseminated gonorrhea Arthritis associated with inflammatory bowel disease Osteoarthritis | ANA, anti-dsDNA, ESR, RF, CBC XR—hands, left knee Cervical culture |

| Presentation | Differential | Workup |
|---|---|---|
| 18 yo M presents with pain in the interphalangeal joints of both hands. He also has scaly, salmon-pink lesions on the extensor surface of his elbows and knees. | **Psoriatic arthritis** <br> Rheumatoid arthritis <br> SLE | RF, ANA, ESR <br> CBC <br> XR—hands |
| 65 yo F presents with inability to use her left leg and bear weight on it after tripping on a carpet. Onset of menopause was 20 years ago, and she did not receive HRT or calcium supplements. Her left leg is externally rotated, shortened, and adducted, and there is tenderness in her left groin. | **Hip fracture** <br> Hip dislocation <br> Pelvic fracture | XR—hip, pelvis <br> CT or MRI—hip <br> CBC |
| 40 yo M presents with pain in the right groin after a motor vehicle accident. His right leg is flexed at the hip, adducted, and internally rotated. | **Hip dislocation—traumatic** <br> Hip fracture | XR—hip <br> CT or MRI—hip <br> CBC |
| 56 yo obese F presents with right knee stiffness and pain that increases with movement. Her symptoms have gradually worsened over the past 10 years. She noticed swelling and deformity of the joint and is having difficulty walking. | **Osteoarthritis** <br> Pseudogout <br> Gout <br> Meniscal or ligament damage | XR—knee <br> CBC <br> ESR <br> Knee arthrocentesis and synovial fluid analysis (cell count, Gram stain, culture, crystals) <br> MRI—knee |
| 45 yo M presents with right knee pain with swelling and redness. | **Septic arthritis** <br> Gout <br> Pseudogout <br> Lyme arthritis <br> Trauma <br> Reiter's arthritis | CBC <br> Knee arthrocentesis and synovial fluid analysis (see above) <br> Blood, urethral cultures <br> XR—knee <br> Uric acid <br> Lyme antibody |
| 65 yo M presents with right foot pain. He has been training for a marathon. | **Stress fracture** <br> Plantar fasciitis <br> Foot sprain or strain | XR—foot <br> Bone scan—foot |

| Presentation | Differential | Workup |
|---|---|---|
| 65 yo M presents with pain in the heel of the right foot that is most notable with his first few steps and then improves as he continues walking. He has no known trauma. | **Plantar fasciitis**<br>Heel fracture<br>Splinter/foreign body | XR—heel<br>Bone scan |
| 55 yo M presents with pain in the elbow when he plays tennis. His grip is impaired as a result of the pain. There is tenderness over the lateral epicondyle as well as pain on resisted wrist dorsiflexion with the elbow in extension. | **Tennis elbow (lateral epicondylitis)**<br>Stress fracture | XR—arm<br>Bone scan<br>MRI—elbow |
| 27 yo F presents with painful wrists and elbows, a swollen and hot knee joint that is painful on flexion, a rash on her limbs, and vaginal discharge. She is sexually active with multiple partners and occasionally uses condoms. | **Disseminated gonorrhea**<br>Rheumatoid arthritis<br>SLE<br>Psoriatic arthritis<br>Reiter's arthritis | Knee arthrocentesis and synovial fluid analysis (cell count, Gram stain, culture)<br>ANA, anti-dsDNA, ESR, RF, CBC<br>Blood, cervical cultures<br>XR—knee |
| 60 yo F presents with pain in both legs that is induced by walking and is relieved by rest. She had cardiac bypass surgery six months ago and continues to smoke heavily. | **Peripheral vascular disease (intermittent claudication)**<br>Leriche's syndrome (aortoiliac occlusive disease)<br>Lumbar spinal stenosis (pseudoclaudication)<br>Osteoarthritis | Doppler U/S—lower<br>Ankle-brachial index<br>Angiography<br>MRI—lumbar spine |
| 45 yo F presents with right calf pain. Her calf is tender, warm, red, and swollen compared to the left side. She was started on OCPs two months ago for dysfunctional uterine bleeding. | **DVT**<br>Baker's cyst rupture<br>Myositis<br>Cellulitis<br>Superficial venous thrombosis | Doppler U/S—right leg<br>CBC<br>CPK<br>D-dimer |
| 50 yo M presents with right shoulder pain after falling onto his outstretched hand while skiing. He noticed deformity of his shoulder and had to hold his right arm. | **Shoulder dislocation**<br>Fracture of the humerus<br>Rotator cuff injury | XR—shoulder<br>XR—arm<br>MRI—shoulder |

MINICASES

93

| Presentation | Differential | Workup |
|---|---|---|
| 55 yo M presents with crampy bilateral thigh and calf pain, fatigue, and dark urine. He is on simvastatin and clofibrate for hyperlipidemia. | **Rhabdomyolysis due to simvastatin or clofibrate** <br> Polymyositis <br> Inclusion body myositis <br> Thyroid disease | CBC <br> CPK <br> Aldolase <br> UA <br> Urine myoglobin <br> TSH |

## ► LOW BACK PAIN

### Key History

Location, quality, intensity, radiation, context (moving furniture, bending/twisting, trauma), timing (disturbs sleep), associated symptoms (especially constitutional, incontinence), exacerbating and alleviating factors; history of cancer, recurrent UTIs, diabetes, renal stones, IV drug use, smoking.

### Key Physical Exam

Vital signs; neurologic exam (especially L4–S1 nerve roots); back palpation and range of motion (although rarely of diagnostic utility); hip exam (can refer pain to the back); consider rectal exam.

| Presentation | Differential | Workup |
|---|---|---|
| 45 yo F presents with low back pain that radiates to the lateral aspect of her left foot. Straight leg raising is positive. The patient is unable to tiptoe. | **Disk herniation** <br> Lumbar muscle strain <br> Tumor in the vertebral canal | XR—L-spine <br> MRI—L-spine |
| 45 yo F presents with low back pain that started after she cleaned her house. The pain does not radiate, and there is no sensory deficit or weakness in her legs. Paraspinal muscle tenderness and spasm are also noted. | **Lumbar muscle strain** <br> Disk herniation <br> Abdominal aortic aneurysm <br> Vertebral compression fracture | XR—L-spine |
| 45 yo M presents with pain in the lower back and legs during prolonged standing and walking. The pain is relieved by sitting and leaning forward (e.g., pushing a grocery cart). | **Lumbar spinal stenosis** <br> Lumbar muscle strain <br> Tumor in the vertebral canal <br> Peripheral vascular disease | XR—L-spine <br> MRI—L-spine (preferred) <br> CT—L-spine <br> Ankle-brachial index |

MINICASES

| Presentation | Differential | Workup |
|---|---|---|
| ▪ 17 yo M presents with low back pain that radiates to the left leg and began after he fell on his knee during gym class. He also describes areas of loss of sensation in his left foot. The pain and sensory loss do not match any known distribution. He insists on requesting a week off from school because of his injury. | **Malingering**<br>Lumbar muscle strain<br>Disk herniation<br>Knee or leg fracture<br>Ankylosing spondylitis | XR—L-spine, knee<br>MRI—L-spine |

(No child will be present; only the mother will be present to tell the story.)

## Key History

Severity, duration, associated localizing symptoms, appetite, rash, sick contacts, day care, immunizations, past history.

## Key Physical Exam

Vital signs; HEENT, neck, heart, lung, abdominal, and skin exams.

| Presentation | Differential | Workup |
|---|---|---|
| ▪ 20-day-old M presents with fever, decreased breast-feeding, and lethargy. He was born at 36 weeks as a result of premature rupture of membranes. | **Neonatal sepsis**<br>Meningitis<br>Pneumonia<br>UTI | Physical exam<br>CBC, electrolytes<br>UA<br>Urine culture<br>Blood culture<br>CXR<br>LP |
| ▪ 3 yo M presents with a two-day history of fever and pulling on his right ear. He is otherwise healthy, and his immunizations are up to date. His older sister recently had a cold. The child attends a day care center. | **Acute otitis media**<br>URI<br>Meningitis<br>UTI | Physical exam (including pneumatic otoscopy)<br>CBC<br>UA |

MINICASES

95

| Presentation | Differential | Workup |
|---|---|---|
| 12-month-old M presents with fever for the last two days accompanied by a maculopapular rash on his face and body. He has not yet received the MMR vaccine. | **Measles (or other viral exanthem)**<br>Rubella<br>Roseola<br>Fifth disease<br>Varicella<br>Scarlet fever<br>Meningitis | Physical exam<br>CBC<br>Viral antibodies/titers<br>Throat swab for culture<br>LP |
| 4 yo M presents with diarrhea, vomiting, lethargy, weakness, and fever. The child attends a day care center where several children have had similar symptoms. | **Gastroenteritis** (viral, bacterial, parasitic)<br>Food poisoning<br>UTI<br>URI<br>Volvulus<br>Intussusception | Physical exam<br>Stool exam and culture<br>CBC<br>Electrolytes<br>UA, urine culture<br>AXR |

MINICASES

# Practice Cases

This chapter consists of 27 commonly encountered cases that approximate those on the actual USMLE Step 2 CS. Each case consists of four parts:

1. **Doorway information sheet:** Designed to simulate the actual information that you will find on the doorway of each examination room, this sheet contains the opening scenario, vital signs, and the tasks you are required to perform during the exam. You should read this sheet just before starting the 15-minute encounter.

2. **Checklist/SP sheet:** This sheet outlines information that standardized patients (SPs) will use to guide them in their encounter and lists questions SPs might ask you, along with potential answers to these questions. Also included is a sample checklist that SPs will use to evaluate your performance.

3. **Blank patient note:** A blank form on which you can write your own note after the patient encounter.

4. **Sample patient note and discussion:** We have included a sample patient note that you can review after you have written your own, as well as a discussion of reasonable differential diagnoses and diagnostic tests to consider in each case.

Because the cases in this section are designed to simulate the actual exam, you can get the most out of them by practicing them with a friend who can act as an SP. To maximize the effectiveness of these practice cases, you should also time each encounter in accordance with the guidelines provided in Sections I and II and compare each of your patient notes with those provided in the text.

For a quicker self-review, you can try to formulate a patient note after reviewing the doorway sheet and the SP checklist and then compare your note with the sample note we have provided.

## Opening Scenario

Sharon Smith, a 48-year-old female, comes to the clinic complaining of abdominal pain.

## Vital Signs

BP: 135/70 mmHg
Temp: 98.5°F (36.9°C)
RR: 16/minute
HR: 76/minute, regular

## Examinee Tasks

1. Take a focused history.
2. Perform a focused physical exam (do not perform rectal, genitourinary, or female breast exam).
3. Explain your clinical impression and workup plan to the patient.
4. Write the patient note after leaving the room.

## Checklist/SP Sheet

PATIENT DESCRIPTION

Patient is a 48 yo F, married with four children.

NOTES FOR THE SP

- Sit up on the bed.
- Show pain on palpation of the right upper abdomen that is exacerbated during inspiration.
- Exhibit epigastric tenderness on palpation.
- If ultrasound is mentioned by the examinee, ask, "What is the meaning of this word?"

CHALLENGING QUESTIONS TO ASK

"My father had pancreatic cancer. Could I have it too?"

SAMPLE EXAMINEE RESPONSE

"It's highly unlikely; your symptoms are very unusual for pancreatic cancer. Regardless, some routine blood and x-ray tests should help us exclude that as a possibility."

## Examinee Checklist

ENTRANCE:

☐ Examinee knocked on the door before entering.
☐ Examinee introduced self by name.
☐ Examinee identified his/her role or position.
☐ Examinee correctly used patient's name.
☐ Examinee made eye contact with the SP.

☐ Examinee showed compassion for your pain.

| ☑ Question | Patient Response |
|---|---|
| ☐ Chief complaint | Abdominal pain. |
| ☐ Onset | Two weeks ago. |
| ☐ Constant/intermittent | Well, I don't have the pain all the time. It comes and goes. |
| ☐ Frequency | At least once every day. |
| ☐ Progression | It is getting worse. |
| ☐ Severity on a scale | When I have the pain, it is 7/10, and then it may go down to 0. |
| ☐ Location | It is here (points to the epigastrium). |
| ☐ Radiation | No. |
| ☐ Quality | Burning. |
| ☐ Alleviating factors | Food, antacids, and milk. |
| ☐ Exacerbating factors | Heavy meals and hunger. |
| ☐ Types of food that exacerbate pain | Heavy, fatty meals, like pizza. |
| ☐ Relationship of food to pain | Well, usually the pain will decrease or stop completely when I eat, but it comes back after 2–3 hours. |
| ☐ Previous episodes of similar pain | No. |
| ☐ Nausea/vomiting | Sometimes I feel nauseated when I am in pain. Yesterday I vomited for the first time. |
| ☐ Description of vomitus | It was a sour, yellowish fluid. |
| ☐ Blood in vomitus | No. |
| ☐ Diarrhea/constipation | No. |
| ☐ Weight changes | No. |
| ☐ Appetite changes | No. |
| ☐ Change in stool color | No. |
| ☐ Current medications | Maalox, ibuprofen (two pills 2–3 times a day if asked). |
| ☐ Past medical history | I had a urinary tract infection one year ago, treated with amoxicillin, and arthritis in both knees. I take ibuprofen for pain. |
| ☐ Past surgical history | I had two C-sections. |
| ☐ Family history | My father died at 55 of pancreatic cancer. My mother is alive and healthy. |
| ☐ Occupation | Housewife. |

| ✓ Question | Patient Response |
|---|---|
| ☐ Alcohol use | No. |
| ☐ Illicit drug use | No. |
| ☐ Tobacco | No. |
| ☐ Sexual activity | With my husband (laughs). |
| ☐ Drug allergies | No. |

## Physical Examination:

- ☐ Examinee washed his/her hands.
- ☐ Examinee asked permission to start the exam.
- ☐ Examinee used respectful draping.
- ☐ Examinee did not repeat painful maneuvers.

| ✓ Exam Component | Maneuver |
|---|---|
| ☐ CV exam | Auscultation |
| ☐ Pulmonary exam | Auscultation |
| ☐ Abdominal exam | Inspection, auscultation, palpation (including Murphy's sign), percussion |

## Closure:

- ☐ Examinee discussed initial diagnostic impressions.
- ☐ Examinee discussed initial management plans:
    - ☐ Follow-up tests: Examinee mentioned the need for a rectal exam.
    - ☐ Examinee asked if the patient has any other questions or concerns.

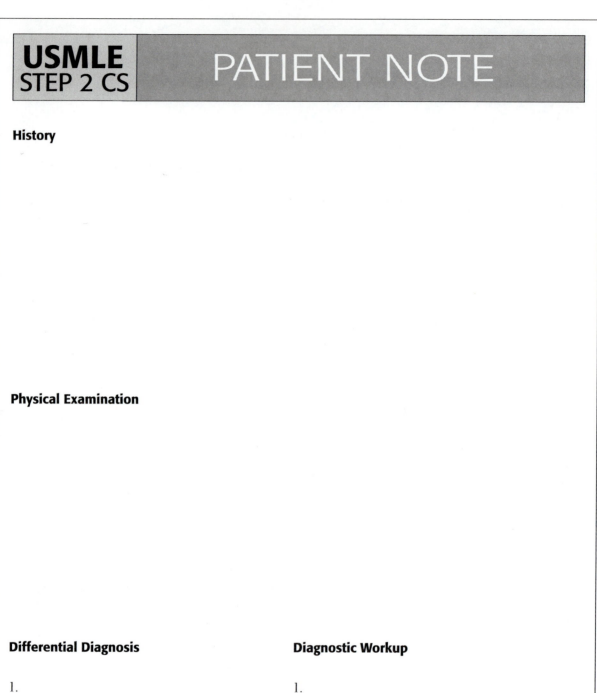

## USMLE STEP 2 CS — PATIENT NOTE

**History**

**Physical Examination**

**Differential Diagnosis**

1.

2.

3.

4.

5.

**Diagnostic Workup**

1.

2.

3.

4.

5.

## History

**HPI:** 48 yo F c/o intermittent, burning, nonradiating epigastric pain that started for the first time 2 weeks ago. The pain occurs at least once a day, usually 2–3 hours after meals. It is exacerbated by hunger and heavy fatty food and is alleviated by milk, antacids, and other food. It reaches 7/10 in severity and then diminishes to 0/10. It is sometimes accompanied by nausea. The patient vomited once yesterday, an acidic yellowish, nonbloody fluid. No diarrhea or constipation. No changes in weight or appetite. No changes in the color of the stool.

**ROS:** Negative except as above.
**Allergies:** NKDA.
**Medications:** Maalox, ibuprofen.
**PMH:** Arthritis in the knees, treated with ibuprofen. UTI last year, treated with amoxicillin.
**PSH:** Two C-sections.
**SH:** No smoking, no EtOH, no illicit drugs. Sexually active with husband only.
**FH:** Father died of pancreatic cancer at age 55.

## Physical Examination

*Patient is in no acute distress.*
**VS:** WNL.
**Chest:** No tenderness, clear breath sounds bilaterally.
**Heart:** RRR; normal S1/S2; no murmurs, rubs, or gallops.
**Abdomen:** Soft, nondistended, C-section scar, epigastric tenderness without rebound, ⊕Murphy's sign, ⊕BS, no hepatosplenomegaly.

## Differential Diagnosis

1. Peptic ulcer disease
2. Cholecystitis
3. Gastritis
4. Functional or nonulcer dyspepsia
5. Perforated ulcer
6. Gastric cancer

## Diagnostic Workup

1. Rectal exam, stool for occult blood
2. AST/ALT/bilirubin/alkaline phosphatase, lipase
3. U/S—abdomen
4. Upper endoscopy
5. HIDA scan
6. *H. pylori* antibody testing

## CASE DISCUSSION

### Differential Diagnosis

Although the causes of abdominal pain are many, this presentation should prompt you to ponder the common etiologies.

- **Peptic ulcer disease:** The history of NSAID use and burning epigastric pain alleviated by antacids and food are consistent with this diagnosis (although the clinical history cannot accurately distinguish duodenal from gastric ulcers).
- **Cholecystitis:** Several features suggest this diagnosis, but the pain in acute cholecystitis is usually unremitting and is not alleviated by milk or antacids. This patient's intermittent pain may be due to "biliary colic," representing transient obstruction of the cystic duct, usually due to gallstones.
- **Gastritis:** This can easily explain epigastric pain, nausea, and vomiting in patients taking NSAIDs.
- **Functional or nonulcer dyspepsia:** This is the most common cause of chronic dyspepsia. After thorough evaluation, no obvious organic etiology is discovered.
- **Perforated ulcer:** These patients appear toxic and have severe diffuse abdominal pain with rebound tenderness and involuntary guarding.
- **Gastric cancer:** Although this patient does not have early satiety, anorexia, weight loss, or a left supraclavicular mass (Virchow's node), it should be noted that signs and symptoms are minimal until late in the course of this rare disease.
- **Other etiologies:** Less likely possibilities include pancreatitis, atypical GERD, choledocholithiasis, mesenteric ischemia, and extra-abdominal causes.

### Diagnostic Workup

- **Rectal exam, stool for occult blood:** May document occult blood loss due to peptic ulcer, gastritis, cancer, or other causes.
- **AST/ALT/bilirubin/alkaline phosphatase, lipase:** To look for evidence of hepatocellular injury, biliary obstruction, or pancreatitis.
- **U/S—abdomen:** A quick, inexpensive imaging technique with which to examine a patient with suspected acute cholecystitis (it may show stones, pericholecystic fluid, a thickened gallbladder wall, and a sonographic Murphy's sign).
- **Upper endoscopy:** Peptic ulcer, gastritis, and gastric cancer have lesions that can be visualized (biopsy is required for gastric cancer diagnosis and sometimes for *H. pylori* diagnosis).
- **HIDA (hepatobiliary) scan:** Can document obstruction of the cystic duct in acute cholecystitis; a positive scan shows absence of filling of the gallbladder. HIDA is usually ordered after U/S (i.e., when the easier but less sensitive U/S does not establish the diagnosis of acute cholecystitis).
- **Noninvasive *H. pylori* testing:** Serologic tests for antibodies to *H. pylori* are adequate for diagnosis but not to document cure, as antibody levels often remain detectable after treatment (indicating exposure, not necessarily active infection). The urease breath test is a useful test with which to confirm *H. pylori* eradication in peptic ulcer disease.

### Opening Scenario

Jessica Anderson, a 21-year-old female, comes to the ER complaining of abdominal pain.

### Vital Signs

**BP:** 120/80 mmHg
**Temp:** 100.5°F (38.1°C)
**RR:** 20/minute
**HR:** 88/minute, regular

### Examinee Tasks

1. Take a focused history.
2. Perform a focused physical exam (do not perform rectal, genitourinary, or female breast exam).
3. Explain your clinical impression and workup plan to the patient.
4. Write the patient note after leaving the room.

### Checklist/SP Sheet

#### PATIENT DESCRIPTION

Patient is a 21 yo F, single with one child.

#### NOTES FOR THE SP

- Exhibit right lower abdominal tenderness on palpation.
- Show rebound tenderness (pain when the examinee removes his palpating hand).
- Demonstrate guarding (contraction of the abdominal muscles when palpating the RLQ).
- Experience pain in the RLQ when the examinee presses on the LLQ (Rovsing's sign).
- Manifest pain when the examinee extends your right hip (psoas sign).

#### CHALLENGING QUESTIONS TO ASK

- "My child is in the house alone. I must leave now."
- "I can't afford to stay in the hospital. Please give me a prescription for antibiotics so that I can leave."

#### SAMPLE EXAMINEE RESPONSE

"First we have to make sure that your illness isn't life-threatening. Our social worker can help us make sure that your child is safe."

### Examinee Checklist

#### ENTRANCE:

☐ Examinee knocked on the door before entering.
☐ Examinee introduced self by name.

☐ Examinee identified his/her role or position.

☐ Examinee correctly used patient's name.

☐ Examinee made eye contact with the SP.

## HISTORY:

☐ Examinee showed compassion for your pain.

| ☑ Question | Patient Response |
| --- | --- |
| ☐ Chief complaint | Abdominal pain. |
| ☐ Onset | This morning. |
| ☐ Frequency | Strong, steady pain. |
| ☐ Progression | It is getting worse. |
| ☐ Severity on a scale | 7/10. |
| ☐ Location | It is here (points to the right lower abdomen). |
| ☐ Radiation | No. |
| ☐ Quality | Cramping. |
| ☐ Alleviating factors | None. |
| ☐ Exacerbating factors | Movement. |
| ☐ Precipitating events | None. |
| ☐ Fever/chills | I've been a little hot since this morning, but no chills. |
| ☐ Nausea/vomiting | I feel nauseated and vomited once two hours ago. |
| ☐ Description of vomitus | It was a sour, yellowish fluid. |
| ☐ Blood in vomitus | No. |
| ☐ Diarrhea/constipation | Loose bowel movements this morning. |
| ☐ Description of stool | Brown. |
| ☐ Blood in stool | No. |
| ☐ Urinary frequency/burning | No. |
| ☐ Last menstrual period | Five weeks ago. |
| ☐ Vaginal spotting | Yes, today is the first day of my menstrual period. |
| ☐ Color of the spotting | Brownish. |
| ☐ Vaginal discharge | No. |
| ☐ Frequency of menstrual periods | Every four weeks; lasts for seven days. |
| ☐ Starting menses | Age 13. |
| ☐ Pads/tampons changed this day | Only one, usually 2–3 a day. |
| ☐ Pregnancies | Three years ago. |

| ☑ **Question** | **Patient Response** |
|---|---|
| ☐ Problems during pregnancy/delivery | No, it was a normal delivery, and my child is healthy. |
| ☐ Miscarriages/abortions | None. |
| ☐ Current medications | Ibuprofen. |
| ☐ Sexual activity | Yes. |
| ☐ Contraceptives | Oral contraceptive pills. My boyfriend refuses to use condoms. |
| ☐ Sexual partners | One partner; I met him two months ago. |
| ☐ Over the last year | I had three sexual partners. |
| ☐ History of STDs | Yes, I had some kind of infection a month ago, but I can't remember the name of it. The doctor gave me a shot and some pills for one week, and then it was over. |
| ☐ Treatment of the partner | He refused the treatment. |
| ☐ HIV test | No. |
| ☐ Past medical history | None except for what I've mentioned. |
| ☐ Past surgical history | None. |
| ☐ Occupation | Waitress. |
| ☐ Alcohol use | Two or three beers a week. |
| ☐ Illicit drug use | No. |
| ☐ Tobacco | One pack a day for the last six years. |
| ☐ Drug allergies | No. |

## Physical Examination:

- ☐ Examinee washed his/her hands.
- ☐ Examinee asked permission to start the exam.
- ☐ Examinee used respectful draping.
- ☐ Examinee did not repeat painful maneuvers.

| ☑ **Exam Component** | **Maneuver** |
|---|---|
| ☐ CV exam | Auscultation |
| ☐ Pulmonary exam | Auscultation |
| ☐ Abdominal exam | Inspection, auscultation, palpation, percussion, psoas sign, obturator sign, Rovsing's sign, CVA tenderness |

## Closure:

- ☐ Examinee discussed initial diagnostic impressions.
- ☐ Examinee discussed initial management plans:

☐ Follow-up tests: Examinee mentioned the need for rectal and pelvic exams.

☐ Discussed safe sex practices.

☐ Counseled regarding smoking cessation.

☐ Offered the assistance of social workers to help the patient identify available financial resources.

☐ Examinee asked if the patient has any other questions or concerns.

**USMLE**
STEP 2 CS

# PATIENT NOTE

**History**

**Physical Examination**

**Differential Diagnosis**

1.
2.
3.
4.
5.

**Diagnostic Workup**

1.
2.
3.
4.
5.

## History

**HPI:** *21 yo G1P1 F c/o right lower abdominal pain that started this morning. The pain is 7/10, crampy, and constant. It is exacerbated by movement and does not radiate. It is accompanied by fever, nausea, vomiting, and loose stools. The patient noticed some brownish spotting this morning. No urinary symptoms; no abnormal vaginal discharge.*
**OB/GYN:** *LMP 5 weeks ago. Regular periods every 4 weeks lasting 7 days. Menarche at age 13. Uncomplicated NSVD (normal spontaneous vaginal delivery) at full term 3 years ago.*
**Allergies:** *NKDA.*
**Medications:** *Ibuprofen.*
**PMH:** *STD 1 month ago, possibly treated with ceftriaxone and doxycycline.*
**PSH:** *None.*
**SH:** *One PPD for 6 years, 2–3 beers/week, no illicit drugs. Unprotected sex with multiple partners.*

## Physical Examination

*Patient is in pain.*
**VS:** *WNL except for temperature of 100.5°F.*
**Chest:** *No tenderness, clear breath sounds bilaterally.*
**Heart:** *RRR; normal S1/S2; no murmurs, rubs, or gallops.*
**Abdomen:** *Soft, nondistended, ⊕BS, no hepatosplenomegaly. Direct and rebound RLQ tenderness, RLQ guarding, ⊕psoas sign, ⊕Rovsing's sign, ⊖obturator sign, no CVA tenderness.*

## Differential Diagnosis

1. PID
2. Appendicitis
3. Ruptured ectopic pregnancy
4. Ruptured ovarian cyst
5. Adnexal torsion
6. Gastroenteritis
7. Abortion
8. Endometriosis

## Diagnostic Workup

1. Rectal exam
2. Pelvic exam
3. Urine hCG
4. Cervical cultures
5. UA
6. CBC
7. U/S—abdomen/pelvis
8. CT—abdomen/pelvis
9. Laparoscopy

## CASE DISCUSSION

### Differential Diagnosis

- **PID:** Suspicion is high for this diagnosis in a patient with multiple sexual partners and a history of STDs who presents with lower abdominal pain and fever. Other findings suggestive of PID include cervical motion tenderness, purulent cervical discharge, adnexal tenderness (usually bilateral), and fever > 101°F (38.3°C).
- **Appendicitis:** Signs and symptoms compatible with this diagnosis are acute right lower abdominal pain that is exacerbated by movement, low-grade fever, nausea, vomiting, direct and rebound RLQ tenderness, RLQ guarding, positive psoas sign, and positive Rovsing's sign.
- **Ruptured ectopic pregnancy:** Even though this patient does not have previously documented PID (or previous tubal pregnancy), the crampy lower abdominal pain, nausea and vomiting, and vaginal spotting occurring after a five-week period of amenorrhea suggest this diagnosis. However, positive psoas and Rovsing's signs are not typical of ectopic pregnancy.
- **Ruptured ovarian cyst:** The sudden-onset unilateral lower abdominal pain, rebound tenderness, and guarding are consistent with this diagnosis. Rupture may occur at any time during the menstrual cycle, and symptoms may resemble a ruptured ectopic pregnancy as described above.
- **Adnexal torsion:** This presentation may be due to adnexal torsion, an uncommon complication that is most often associated with ovarian enlargement due to a benign mass.
- **Gastroenteritis:** Viral gastroenteritis presents with crampy abdominal pain, nausea and vomiting, low-grade fever, and diarrhea. It can be difficult to distinguish from appendicitis and gynecologic etiologies but is less likely in this case given the presence of rebound tenderness.
- **Abortion:** The fact that the patient's last menstrual period was only five weeks ago makes this less likely, but the crampy abdominal pain and vaginal spotting may signal an abortion. Furthermore, the presence of fever suggests possible septic abortion.
- **Endometriosis:** This is an unlikely diagnosis, in part because the patient has no history of chronic pelvic pain, dysmenorrhea, dyspareunia, or infertility, which are often associated. In a patient with established endometriosis, this presentation with acute severe pain, including rebound tenderness, could be due to rupture of an endometrioma ("chocolate cyst").

### Diagnostic Workup

- **Rectal exam:** Elicits pain on the right side of the abdomen in acute appendicitis (not very specific).
- **Pelvic exam:** Look for cervical motion tenderness and discharge, uterine size, and adnexal masses or tenderness.
- **Urine hCG:** Positive in pregnancy. Urine and serum tests are equally sensitive, but obtaining quantitative hCG levels (available only via serum test) may help diagnose and treat ectopic pregnancy.
- **Cervical cultures:** *Neisseria gonorrhoeae* and *Chlamydia trachomatis*, the main causes of PID, are detected via DNA probes.
- **UA:** To rule out UTI.
- **CBC:** Findings are nonspecific, but can see leukocytosis in infection or appendicitis.
- **U/S–abdomen/pelvis:** Can help diagnose appendiceal or ovarian pathology. Transvaginal U/S can identify an intrauterine gestational sac when the time elapsed since the last menstrual period is 35 days (this corresponds to a $\beta$-hCG of about 1500); fluid in the cul-de-sac is nonspecific and may suggest ectopic pregnancy or a ruptured ovarian cyst.
- **CT–abdomen/pelvis:** Can detect the presence of appendiceal inflammation, abscess in appendicitis, or signs of other GI or gynecologic pathology.
- **Laparoscopy:** Can diagnose ectopic pregnancy (gold standard), ruptured ovarian cyst, ovarian torsion, PID ± tubo-ovarian abscess, appendicitis, etc.

### Opening Scenario

Richard Green, a 74-year-old male, comes to the ER complaining of pain in his right arm.

### Vital Signs

BP: 135/85 mmHg
Temp: 98.0°F (36.7°C)
RR: 12/minute
HR: 76/minute, regular

### Examinee Tasks

1. Take a focused history.
2. Perform a focused physical exam (do not perform rectal, genitourinary, or female breast exam).
3. Explain your clinical impression and workup plan to the patient.
4. Write the patient note after leaving the room.

### Checklist/SP Sheet

PATIENT DESCRIPTION

Patient is a 74 yo M.

NOTES FOR THE SP

- Sit up on the bed.
- Hold your right arm close to your body with your left hand and keep it internally rotated.
- Show pain when the examinee tries to move your right shoulder in any direction.
- Do not allow the examinee to bring your shoulder to its full range of motion in flexion, extension, abduction, or external rotation.

CHALLENGING QUESTIONS TO ASK

"Doctor, do you think I will be able to move my arm again like before?"

SAMPLE EXAMINEE RESPONSE

"I hope so, but first we need to confirm whether it's broken or dislocated and whether there is any nerve or muscle damage."

### Examinee Checklist

ENTRANCE:

☐ Examinee knocked on the door before entering.
☐ Examinee introduced self by name.
☐ Examinee identified his/her role or position.

☐ Examinee correctly used patient's name.

☐ Examinee made eye contact with the SP.

## HISTORY:

☐ Examinee showed compassion for your pain.

| ☑ Question | Patient Response |
|---|---|
| ☐ Chief complaint | Pain in the right arm. |
| ☐ Onset | Three days ago. |
| ☐ Precipitating events | I was playing with my grandchildren in the garden when I tripped and fell. |
| ☐ Description of the fall | I tripped over a toy on the ground and fell on my hand. My arm was outstretched. |
| ☐ Loss of consciousness | No. |
| ☐ Location | The upper and middle parts of the arm. |
| ☐ Weakness/paralysis | None. |
| ☐ Numbness/loss of sensation | None. |
| ☐ Progression of pain | I didn't feel any pain at the time, and then the pain started gradually. It is stable now, but it is still there. |
| ☐ Pain anywhere else | No. |
| ☐ Seen by a doctor since then | No. |
| ☐ Any treatments | I used a sling and took some Tylenol, but the pain didn't get better. |
| ☐ Alleviating factors | Not moving my arm and Tylenol. |
| ☐ Exacerbating factors | Moving my arm. |
| ☐ Reason for not seeking medical attention | Well, it wasn't that bad, and I thought it would get better on its own (looks anxious). Also, my son didn't have time to bring me to the hospital; he was busy. |
| ☐ Living conditions | I live with my son. He is married and has three children. Life has been hard on him lately. He lost his job and is looking for a new one. |
| ☐ Social history | I am a widower; my wife died three years ago, and since then I've lived with my son. |
| ☐ Bad treatment in his son's house | No (looks anxious). They are all nice. |
| ☐ Current medications | Tylenol, albuterol inhaler. |
| ☐ Allergies | Yes, I am allergic to aspirin. |
| ☐ Past medical history | Asthma. |

| ☑ *Question* | *Patient Response* |
|---|---|
| ☐ Past surgical history | They removed my prostate two years ago. It was very difficult for me to urinate, but that has gotten much better. They said there was no evidence of cancer. |
| ☐ Occupation | Retired schoolteacher. |
| ☐ Alcohol use | No. |
| ☐ Tobacco | No. |
| ☐ Exercise | Every day I walk for 20 minutes to the grocery store and back. |

## Physical Examination:

☐ Examinee washed his/her hands.
☐ Examinee asked permission to start the exam.
☐ Examinee used respectful draping.
☐ Examinee did not repeat painful maneuvers.

| ☑ *Exam Component* | *Maneuver* |
|---|---|
| ☐ Head and neck exam | Checked for bruises, neck movements |
| ☐ CV exam | Auscultation |
| ☐ Pulmonary exam | Auscultation |
| ☐ Exam of the arms | Compared both arms in terms of strength, range of motion (shoulder, elbow, wrist), sensation, DTRs, pulses |

## Closure:

☐ Examinee discussed initial diagnostic impressions.
☐ Examinee discussed initial management plans:
    ☐ Diagnostic tests.
    ☐ Discussed alternative living options such as assisted living.
    ☐ Offered social work assistance.
    ☐ Offered a statement of support: "Your safety is my primary concern, and I am here for help and support when you need it."
☐ Examinee asked if the patient has any other questions or concerns.

**USMLE STEP 2 CS** PATIENT NOTE

**History**

**Physical Examination**

**Differential Diagnosis**

1.
2.
3.
4.
5.

**Diagnostic Workup**

1.
2.
3.
4.
5.

## History

**HPI:** 74 yo M c/o pain in the right arm. The pain started 3 days ago, after he fell on his outstretched right hand. Treated at home with Tylenol and a sling, but pain persisted. No loss of consciousness before or after the fall. No paralysis or loss of sensation. The pain is in the upper and middle part of the arm, increases with any movement of the arm, and is alleviated by Tylenol and rest. When asked about the reason for the delay in seeking medical assistance, the patient looked anxious and stated that his son didn't have time to take him to the hospital.

**ROS:** Negative except as above.

**Allergies:** Aspirin.

**Medications:** Tylenol, albuterol inhaler.

**PMH:** Asthma, probable BPH s/p prostate surgery.

**SH:** No smoking, no EtOH. Widower for the last 3 years; lives with his son, who recently lost his job. Walks 20 minutes every morning.

## Physical Examination

Patient is in no acute distress.

**VS:** WNL.

**HEENT:** Normocephalic, atraumatic, no bruises.

**Neck:** Supple, full range of motion in all directions, no bruises.

**Chest:** Clear breath sounds bilaterally.

**Heart:** RRR; normal S1/S2; no murmurs, rubs, or gallops.

**Extremities:** Tenderness over the middle and upper right arm and the right shoulder; pain and restricted range of motion on flexion, extension, abduction, and external rotation of the right shoulder. Right elbow and wrist are normal. Pulses normal and symmetric in brachial and radial arteries. Unable to assess muscle strength due to pain. DTRs intact and symmetric. Sensation intact to pinprick and soft touch.

## Differential Diagnosis

1. Humeral fracture
2. Osteoporosis
3. Shoulder dislocation
4. Elder abuse
5. Rotator cuff tear

## Diagnostic Workup

1. XR—right shoulder and arm
2. MRI—shoulder
3. Bone density scan (DEXA)

## CASE DISCUSSION

### Differential Diagnosis

- **Humeral fracture:** Occurs most commonly in elderly persons, usually after a fall. The axillary nerve can be injured in a proximal humerus fracture, causing sensory loss along the lateral aspect of the deltoid region. The radial nerve can be injured in a fracture of the midshaft/distal third of the humerus, causing wrist drop.
- **Osteoporosis:** Suspect underlying osteoporosis in elderly patients (especially women) presenting with fractures following minimal trauma. The most common sites of osteoporotic fractures are the thoracic and lumbar vertebral bodies, the neck of the femur, and the distal radius.
- **Shoulder dislocation:** The glenohumeral joint is the most commonly dislocated joint in the human body. It most often dislocates anteriorly and usually results from a fall on an outstretched hand with forceful abduction, extension, and external rotation of the shoulder. On exam the arm is held in the neutral position, and movement is avoided owing to pain.
- **Elder abuse:** The history contains red flags (bruises, anxious behavior) that may indicate elder abuse. The American Medical Association has defined elder abuse as "an act or omission which results in harm or threatened harm to the health or welfare of an elderly person." The diagnosis of elder abuse is not readily made because more often than not, both the abuser and the victim may deny abuse. Thus, diagnosis is inferential in many cases, and supporting evidence must be sought.
- **Rotator cuff tear:** Patients usually present with nonspecific pain localized to the shoulder, but pain is often referred down the proximal lateral arm owing to shared innervation. There may be an inability to abduct or flex the shoulder.

### Diagnostic Workup

- **XR—right shoulder and arm:** AP and lateral views that include the joints above and below the injury can show fracture or dislocation. An axillary view is useful to help diagnose proximal humeral fracture or dislocation.
- **MRI—shoulder:** Required to diagnose rotator cuff tears, labral disease, and other disorders.
- **Bone density scan (DEXA):** To diagnose and quantify osteoporosis.

# CASE 4

## DOORWAY INFORMATION

### Opening Scenario

Brian Davis, a 21-year-old male, comes to the office complaining of a sore throat.

### Vital Signs

**BP:** 120/80 mmHg
**Temp:** 99.5°F (37.5°C)
**RR:** 15/minute
**HR:** 75/minute, regular

### Examinee Tasks

1. Take a focused history.
2. Perform a focused physical exam (do not perform rectal, genitourinary, or female breast exam).
3. Explain your clinical impression and workup plan to the patient.
4. Write the patient note after leaving the room.

### Checklist/SP Sheet

PATIENT DESCRIPTION

Patient is a 21 yo M.

NOTES FOR THE SP

- Be rude and defensive.
- Make most of your answers a curt "yes" or "no."
- Pretend that you have LUQ tenderness on abdominal palpation.

CHALLENGING QUESTIONS TO ASK

"Do you think I have AIDS?"

SAMPLE EXAMINEE RESPONSE

"That's a difficult question; first I need to find out why you are so concerned about AIDS. Have you been exposed to HIV infection?"

### Examinee Checklist

ENTRANCE:

- ☐ Examinee knocked on the door before entering.
- ☐ Examinee introduced self by name.
- ☐ Examinee identified his/her role or position.
- ☐ Examinee correctly used patient's name.
- ☐ Examinee made eye contact with the SP.

☐ Examinee showed compassion for your illness.

| ☑ Question | Patient Response |
| --- | --- |
| ☐ Chief complaint | Sore throat. |
| ☐ Onset | Two weeks ago. |
| ☐ Runny nose | No. |
| ☐ Fever/chills | Mild fever over the last two weeks, but I didn't take my temperature. No chills. |
| ☐ Night sweats | No. |
| ☐ Cough | No. |
| ☐ Swollen glands and lymph nodes | Yes, in my neck (if asked); a little painful (if asked). |
| ☐ Jaundice | No. |
| ☐ Chest pain | No. |
| ☐ Shortness of breath | No. |
| ☐ Abdominal pain | I've had some discomfort here (points to LUQ) constantly since yesterday. |
| ☐ Radiation | No. |
| ☐ Severity on a scale | 4/10. |
| ☐ Relationship of food to pain | No. |
| ☐ Alleviating/exacerbating factors | No. |
| ☐ Nausea/vomiting | No. |
| ☐ Change in bowel habits | No. |
| ☐ Change in urinary habits | No. |
| ☐ Headache | No. |
| ☐ Fatigue | I have been feeling tired for the past two weeks. |
| ☐ Ill contacts | My ex-girlfriend had the same thing two months ago. I don't know what happened to her, because we broke up when she got sick. |
| ☐ Changes in weight | Yes, I feel that I am losing weight, but I don't know how much. |
| ☐ Appetite changes | I don't feel like eating anything at all. |
| ☐ Current medications | Tylenol. |
| ☐ Past medical history | I had gonorrhea four months ago. I took some antibiotics. |
| ☐ Past surgical history | None. |
| ☐ Family history | My father and mother are alive and in good health. |

| ☑ Question | Patient Response |
|---|---|
| ☐ Occupation | Last year in college. |
| ☐ Alcohol use | Yes, on the weekends. |
| ☐ Illicit drug use | No. |
| ☐ Tobacco | Yes, I smoke one pack a day. I started when I was 15 years old. |
| ☐ Sexual activity | I have a new girlfriend. |
| ☐ Use of condoms | Yes. |
| ☐ Active with men, women, or both | Men and women. |
| ☐ Number of sexual partners during the last year | Two. |
| ☐ History of STDs | I told you, I had gonorrhea four months ago, and I was cured after a course of antibiotics. |
| ☐ Drug allergies | No. |

## Physical Examination:

☐ Examinee washed his/her hands.
☐ Examinee asked permission to start the exam.
☐ Examinee used respectful draping.
☐ Examinee did not repeat painful maneuvers.

| ☑ Exam Component | Maneuver |
|---|---|
| ☐ Head and neck exam | Examined nose, mouth, throat, lymph nodes; checked for sinus tenderness |
| ☐ CV exam | Auscultation |
| ☐ Pulmonary exam | Auscultation |
| ☐ Abdominal exam | Auscultation, palpation, percussion |

## Closure:

☐ Examinee discussed initial diagnostic impressions.
☐ Examinee discussed initial management plans:
    ☐ Follow-up tests (including consent for HIV testing).
    ☐ Discussed safe sex practices.
    ☐ Counseled to avoid contact sports in light of possible increased risk of traumatic splenic rupture.
    ☐ Examinee asked if the patient has any other questions or concerns.

**USMLE**
STEP 2 CS

# PATIENT NOTE

**History**

**Physical Examination**

**Differential Diagnosis**

1.
2.
3.
4.
5.

**Diagnostic Workup**

1.
2.
3.
4.
5.

## History

**HPI:** *21 yo M c/o sore throat for the last 2 weeks. Two weeks ago he had a mild fever and fatigue, but he denies any chills, runny nose, cough, night sweats, shortness of breath, or wheezing. The patient also notes LUQ abdominal pain since yesterday. The pain is 4/10 and constant with no radiation, no relation to food, and no alleviating or exacerbating factors. He has poor appetite and subjective weight loss. His ex-girlfriend had the same symptoms 2 months ago.*
**ROS:** *Negative except as above.*
**Allergies:** *NKDA.*
**Medications:** *Tylenol.*
**PMH:** *Gonorrhea 4 months ago, treated with antibiotics.*
**SH:** *One PPD since age 15; drinks heavily on weekends. Multiple female and male partners; uses condoms.*
**FH:** *Noncontributory.*

## Physical Examination

*Patient is in no acute distress.*
**VS:** *WNL.*
**HEENT:** *Nose, mouth, and pharynx WNL.*
**Neck:** *Supple, no lymphadenopathy.*
**Chest:** *Clear breath sounds bilaterally.*
**Heart:** *RRR; normal S1/S2; no murmurs, rubs, or gallops.*
**Abdomen:** *Soft, nondistended, ⊕BS, no hepatosplenomegaly, mild LUQ tenderness on palpation.*
**Skin:** *No rash.*

## Differential Diagnosis

1. Infectious mononucleosis
2. Acute HIV infection
3. Viral pharyngitis
4. Bacterial pharyngitis

## Diagnostic Workup

1. CBC
2. Peripheral smear
3. Monospot
4. Rapid streptococcal antigen
5. Throat culture
6. Anti-EBV antibodies
7. HIV antibody and viral load

## CASE DISCUSSION

### Differential Diagnosis

- **Infectious mononucleosis:** The differential diagnosis for "sore throat" includes many pathogens. This patient's LUQ pain suggests splenomegaly, which could limit the differential (for a unifying diagnosis) to an infectious mononucleosis caused by EBV or, less commonly, by CMV infection. Recall that the physical exam is notoriously insensitive for detecting splenomegaly and may be misleading, as in this case. However, this patient does not have other typical features of infectious mononucleosis, such as lymphadenopathy or exudative pharyngitis.
- **Group A streptococcal pharyngitis:** Clinical features in patients with sore throat that predict group A streptococcal pharyngitis include tonsillar exudates, tender anterior cervical lymphadenopathy, a history of fever (temperature > 100.4°F/38°C), and absence of cough. "Strep throat" must be recognized and treated in order to prevent acute rheumatic fever.
- **Other common etiologies:** Include viruses (including acute HIV infection, which is often associated with a generalized maculopapular rash), *Neisseria gonorrhoeae*, *Mycoplasma* (although lower respiratory symptoms usually predominate), rubella, and *Chlamydia trachomatis*.

### Diagnostic Workup

- **CBC:** Findings are nonspecific, but can see leukocytosis in infection.
- **Peripheral smear:** Can reveal atypical lymphocytes in infectious mononucleosis.
- **Monospot (heterophil agglutination test):** Usually becomes positive in EBV-associated mononucleosis within four weeks of onset of illness.
- **Rapid streptococcal antigen:** Has high negative predictive value (i.e., it can accurately confirm the absence of group A streptococcal pharyngitis).
- **Throat culture:** The gold standard for diagnosing bacterial pharyngitis.
- **Anti-EBV antibodies:** Antibodies to various EBV antigens can be detected, such as IgM antibody to virus capsid antigen (VCA) and to nuclear antigen (EBNA). There is also a PCR to detect EBV in serum.
- **HIV antibody and viral load:** Check antibody to exclude preexisting HIV infection, and check viral load to help document acute infection.

## DOORWAY INFORMATION

### Opening Scenario

Kenneth Klein, a 55-year-old male, comes to the clinic complaining of blood in his stool.

### Vital Signs

BP: 130/80 mmHg
Temp: 98.5°F (36.9°C)
RR: 16/minute
HR: 76/minute, regular

### Examinee Tasks

1. Take a focused history.
2. Perform a focused physical exam (do not perform rectal, genitourinary, or female breast exams).
3. Explain your clinical impression and workup plan to the patient.
4. Write the patient note after leaving the room.

### Checklist/SP Sheet

PATIENT DESCRIPTION

Patient is a 55 yo M, married with two children.

NOTES FOR THE SP

If colonoscopy is mentioned by the examinee, ask, "What is the meaning of this word?"

CHALLENGING QUESTIONS TO ASK

"My father had colon cancer. Could I have it too?"

SAMPLE EXAMINEE RESPONSE

"It is a possibility. Tell me more about the symptoms you're having that concern you with regard to cancer."

### Examinee Checklist

ENTRANCE:

☐ Examinee knocked on the door before entering.
☐ Examinee introduced self by name.
☐ Examinee identified his/her role or position.
☐ Examinee correctly used patient's name.
☐ Examinee made eye contact with the SP.

HISTORY:

☐ Examinee showed compassion for your illness.

| ☑ Question | Patient Response |
|---|---|
| ☐ Chief complaint | Blood in stool. |
| ☐ Onset | One month ago. |
| ☐ Frequency | Every time I move my bowels, I see some blood mixed in with the stool. |
| ☐ Description (blood before, during, or after defecation) | The blood is mixed in with the brown stool. |
| ☐ Pain during defecation | No. |
| ☐ Constipation | Well, I have had constipation for a long time, and I keep taking laxatives. At first I used to get some relief, but now there is no benefit from them. |
| ☐ Frequency of bowel movements | I have had two bowel movements a week for the last six months. |
| ☐ Diarrhea | I have had diarrhea for the past two days. |
| ☐ Urgency | No. |
| ☐ Tenesmus (ineffectual spasms of the rectum, accompanied by the desire to empty the bowel) | A little. |
| ☐ Frequency of diarrhea | Three times a day. |
| ☐ Description of the diarrhea | Watery, brown, mixed with blood. |
| ☐ Mucus in stool | No. |
| ☐ Melena | No. |
| ☐ Fever/chills | No. |
| ☐ Abdominal pain | No. |
| ☐ Nausea/vomiting | No. |
| ☐ Diet | I eat a lot of junk food. I don't eat vegetables at all. |
| ☐ Weight changes | I have lost about 10 pounds over the past six months. |
| ☐ Appetite changes | My appetite has been the same. |
| ☐ Recent travel | No, but I am thinking of going on a trip with my family next week. Do you think I should stay home? |
| ☐ Contact with people with diarrhea | No. |
| ☐ Exercise | I walk for half an hour every day. |
| ☐ Urinary problems | No. |
| ☐ Current medications | No. I used to take many laxatives, such as bisacodyl and phenolphthalein, but I stopped all of them when the diarrhea started. |
| ☐ Past medical history | I had bronchitis three weeks ago; treated with amoxicillin. |
| ☐ Past surgical history | Hemorrhoids resected four years ago. |

| ✓ Question | Patient Response |
|---|---|
| ☐ Family history | My father died at 55 of colon cancer. My mother is alive and healthy. |
| ☐ Occupation | Lawyer. |
| ☐ Alcohol use | No. |
| ☐ Illicit drug use | No. |
| ☐ Tobacco | No. |
| ☐ Sexual activity | With my wife. |
| ☐ Drug allergies | None. |

## Physical Examination:

☐ Examinee washed his/her hands.

☐ Examinee asked permission to start the exam.

☐ Examinee used respectful draping.

☐ Examinee did not repeat painful maneuvers.

| ✓ Exam Component | Maneuver |
|---|---|
| ☐ CV exam | Auscultation |
| ☐ Pulmonary exam | Auscultation |
| ☐ Abdominal exam | Auscultation, palpation, percussion |

## Closure:

☐ Examinee discussed initial diagnostic impressions.

☐ Examinee discussed initial management plans:

    ☐ Follow-up tests: Examinee mentioned the need for a rectal exam.

☐ Examinee asked if the patient has any other questions or concerns.

**USMLE**
STEP 2 CS

# PATIENT NOTE

**History**

**Physical Examination**

**Differential Diagnosis**

1.
2.
3.
4.
5.

**Diagnostic Workup**

1.
2.
3.
4.
5.

## History

**HPI:** 55 yo M c/o blood in stool. He has a history of constipation that started 6 months ago, consisting of 2 bowel movements a week. One month ago he noticed blood mixed with stool at every bowel movement. During the last 2 days he started to have tenesmus and watery brown diarrhea (3 times a day) mixed with blood. He has no urgency, no mucus in stool, and no pain during defecation. He denies any fever, chills, nausea, vomiting, abdominal pain, recent history of travel, or contact with ill persons. He recalls a 10-pound weight loss during the last 6 months despite a good appetite. His diet consists of a lot of junk food with no vegetables.
**ROS:** Negative except as above.
**Allergies:** NKDA.
**Medications:** Used to take many laxatives (bisacodyl, phenolphthalein) but stopped after the onset of diarrhea 2 days ago.
**PMH:** Bronchitis 3 weeks ago, treated with amoxicillin.
**PSH:** Hemorrhoids resected 4 years ago.
**SH:** No smoking, no EtOH, no illicit drugs. Sexually active with wife only.
**FH:** Father died of colon cancer at age 55.

## Physical Examination

Patient is in no acute distress.
**VS:** WNL.
**Chest:** Clear breath sounds bilaterally.
**Heart:** RRR; normal S1/S2; no murmurs, rubs, or gallops.
**Abdomen:** Soft, nondistended, nontender, ⊕BS, no hepatosplenomegaly.

## Differential Diagnosis

1. Colorectal cancer
2. Hemorrhoids
3. Diverticulosis
4. Angiodysplasia
5. Pseudomembranous (C. difficile) colitis
6. Other infectious colitis
7. Ulcerative colitis

## Diagnostic Workup

1. Rectal exam, stool for occult blood
2. Stool for C. difficile toxin
3. Fecal leukocytes
4. CBC
5. Anoscopy
6. Flexible proctosigmoidoscopy
7. Colonoscopy
8. Double-contrast (air contrast) barium enema
9. CT—abdomen/pelvis

# CASE DISCUSSION

## Differential Diagnosis

Bright red blood that is mixed with brown stool suggests a distal colonic or anorectal source. Otherwise, this patient's presentation is complex, and the differential remains broad. His chronic constipation may simply be due to a low-fiber diet or to irritable bowel syndrome, but neither of these entities explains hematochezia and weight loss.

- **Colorectal cancer:** A positive family history coupled with the presence of blood in the stool, a change in bowel habits, and weight loss makes colorectal cancer a plausible diagnosis. Screening colonoscopy should have been offered to the patient at age 45 (10 years prior to the age when a first-degree family member was diagnosed).
- **Hemorrhoids:** Recurrent hemorrhoids may explain the patient's hematochezia, although more typical findings in hemorrhoids are fresh blood on the paper or dripped into the toilet bowl.
- **Diverticulosis:** This is the most common cause of major lower GI bleeding, but it usually presents with larger-volume bleeds occurring in discrete, self-limited episodes.
- **Angiodysplasia:** This is another common cause of lower GI tract bleeding, but as with diverticular disease, it cannot explain the other features of this patient's presentation.
- **Pseudomembranous (*C. difficile*) colitis:** It is important to ask all patients with acute diarrhea about recent antibiotic exposure, as symptoms of antibiotic-associated colitis may be delayed for up to 6–8 weeks. Stools rarely contain gross blood, however. The absence of fever and lower abdominal cramping also makes this diagnosis (and other infectious colitis) less likely.
- **Ulcerative colitis:** The absence of abdominal pain and the very recent onset of diarrhea and tenesmus make inflammatory bowel disease a less likely etiology for this patient's month-long hematochezia.

## Diagnostic Workup

- **Rectal exam, stool for occult blood:** Useful to detect masses and hemorrhoids. Always test for occult blood in stool.
- **Stool for *C. difficile* toxin:** Recall that one negative test does not exclude the diagnosis, as the assays are positive in only 80% of patients on the first stool sample and in 90% after two stool samples.
- **Fecal leukocytes:** Usually present in invasive bacterial infection and in inflammatory bowel disease. Variably present in *C. difficile* colitis.
- **CBC:** To investigate anemia. Also, leukocytosis could suggest infection or inflammatory bowel disease.
- **Anoscopy:** Can identify bleeding internal hemorrhoids, rectal ulcers, and traumatic lesions.
- **Flexible proctosigmoidoscopy:** If nondiagnostic, follow up with a barium enema or a colonoscopy.
- **Colonoscopy:** Should be the initial test performed in patients > 40 years of age presenting with hematochezia.
- **Double-contrast (air contrast) barium enema:** Not as accurate as colonoscopy for the diagnosis of polyps and cancer (and cannot diagnose angiodysplasia). Used mainly when colonoscopy is unavailable or contraindicated.
- **CT–abdomen/pelvis:** Contrast-enhanced exams can detect diverticulosis or masses but generally are not useful in the evaluation of GI bleeding.

# CASE 6

## DOORWAY INFORMATION

### Opening Scenario

Joseph Short, a 46-year-old male, comes to the ER complaining of chest pain.

### Vital Signs

**BP:** 165/85 mmHg
**Temp:** 98.6°F (37°C)
**RR:** 22/minute
**HR:** 90/minute, regular

### Examinee Tasks

1. Take a focused history.
2. Perform a focused physical exam (do not perform rectal, genitourinary, or female breast exams).
3. Explain your clinical impression and workup plan to the patient.
4. Write the patient note after leaving the room.

### Checklist/SP Sheet

PATIENT DESCRIPTION

Patient is a 46 yo M.

NOTES FOR THE SP

- Lie on the bed and exhibit pain.
- Place your hands in the middle of your chest.
- Exhibit difficulty breathing.
- If ECG is mentioned by the examinee, ask, "What is an ECG?"

CHALLENGING QUESTIONS TO ASK

"Is this a heart attack? Am I going to die?"

SAMPLE EXAMINEE RESPONSE

"As you suspect, your symptoms are of considerable concern. We need to learn more about what's going on to know if your pain is life-threatening."

### Examinee Checklist

ENTRANCE:

☐ Examinee knocked on the door before entering.
☐ Examinee introduced self by name.
☐ Examinee identified his/her role or position.
☐ Examinee correctly used patient's name.
☐ Examinee made eye contact with the SP.

☐ Examinee showed compassion for your pain.

| ☑ **Question** | **Patient Response** |
|---|---|
| ☐ Chief complaint | Chest pain. |
| ☐ Onset | Forty minutes ago. |
| ☐ Precipitating events | Nothing; I was asleep and I woke up at 5:00 in the morning having this pain. |
| ☐ Progression | Constant severity. |
| ☐ Severity on a scale | 7/10. |
| ☐ Location | Middle of the chest. |
| ☐ Radiation | To my neck and left arm. |
| ☐ Quality | Pressure. |
| ☐ Alleviating/exacerbating factors | Nothing. |
| ☐ Shortness of breath | Yes. |
| ☐ Nausea/vomiting | I feel nauseated, but I didn't vomit. |
| ☐ Sweating | Yes. |
| ☐ Associated symptoms (cough, wheezing, abdominal pain, diarrhea/constipation) | None. |
| ☐ Previous episodes of similar pain | Yes, but not exactly the same. |
| ☐ Onset | Past three months. |
| ☐ Severity | Less severe. |
| ☐ Frequency | Two to three episodes a week. |
| ☐ Precipitating events | Walking up the stairs, strenuous work, and heavy meals. |
| ☐ Alleviating factors | Antacids. |
| ☐ Associated symptoms | None. |
| ☐ Current medications | Maalox, diuretic. |
| ☐ Past medical history | Hypertension for five years, treated with a diuretic. High cholesterol, managed with diet; I have not been very compliant with the diet. GERD 10 years ago, treated with antacids. |
| ☐ Past surgical history | None. |
| ☐ Family history | My father died of lung cancer. My mother is alive and has a peptic ulcer. No early heart attacks. |
| ☐ Occupation | Accountant. |
| ☐ Alcohol use | Once in a while. |
| ☐ Illicit drug use | Cocaine, once a week. |

| ☑ Question | Patient Response |
|---|---|
| ☐ Last time of cocaine use | Yesterday afternoon. |
| ☐ Tobacco | Stopped three months ago. |
| ☐ Duration | Twenty-five years. |
| ☐ Amount | One pack a day. |
| ☐ Sexual activity | Well, doctor, to be honest, I haven't had sex with my wife for the last three months, because I get this pain in my chest during sex. |
| ☐ Exercise | No. |
| ☐ Diet | My doctor gave me a strict diet last year to lower my cholesterol, but I always cheat. |
| ☐ Drug allergies | No. |

## Physical Examination:

- ☐ Examinee washed his/her hands.
- ☐ Examinee asked permission to start the exam.
- ☐ Examinee used respectful draping.
- ☐ Examinee did not repeat painful maneuvers.

| ☑ Exam Component | Maneuver |
|---|---|
| ☐ Neck exam | Looked for JVD, carotid auscultation |
| ☐ CV exam | Inspection, palpation, auscultation |
| ☐ Pulmonary exam | Auscultation, palpation, percussion |
| ☐ Abdominal exam | Auscultation, palpation, percussion |
| ☐ Extremities | Checked peripheral pulses, checked blood pressure in both arms, looked for edema |

## Closure:

- ☐ Examinee discussed initial diagnostic impressions.
- ☐ Examinee discussed initial management plans:
    - ☐ Diagnostic tests.
    - ☐ Lifestyle modification (diet, exercise).
- ☐ Examinee asked if the patient has any other questions or concerns.

**USMLE STEP 2 CS** PATIENT NOTE

**History**

**Physical Examination**

**Differential Diagnosis**

1.
2.
3.
4.
5.

**Diagnostic Workup**

1.
2.
3.
4.
5.

### History

**HPI:** 46 yo M c/o chest pain. Chest pain started 40 minutes before the patient presented to the ER. The pain woke the patient from sleep at 5 A.M. with a steady 7/10 pressure sensation in the middle of his chest that radiated to the left arm and the neck. Nothing makes it worse or better. Nausea, sweating, and dyspnea are also present. Similar episodes have occurred during the past 3 months, 2–3 times/week. These episodes were precipitated by walking up the stairs, strenuous work, sexual intercourse, and heavy meals. Pain during these episodes was less severe, lasted for 5–10 minutes, and disappeared spontaneously or after taking antacids.

**ROS:** Negative except as above.

**Allergies:** NKDA.

**Medications:** Maalox, diuretic.

**PMH:** Hypertension for 5 years, treated with a diuretic. High cholesterol, managed with diet. GERD 10 years ago, treated with antacids.

**SH:** One PPD for 25 years; stopped 3 months ago. Occasional EtOH, occasional cocaine (last used yesterday afternoon). No regular exercise; poorly adherent to diet.

**FH:** Father died of lung cancer at age 72. Mother has peptic ulcers. No early coronary disease.

### Physical Examination

*Patient is in severe pain.*

**VS:** BP 165/85 (both arms), RR 22.

**Neck:** No JVD, no bruits.

**Chest:** No tenderness, clear symmetric breath sounds bilaterally.

**Heart:** Apical impulse not displaced; RRR; normal S1/S2; no murmurs, rubs, or gallops.

**Abdomen:** Soft, nondistended, nontender, ⊕BS, no hepatosplenomegaly.

**Extremities:** No edema, peripheral pulses 2+ and symmetric.

### Differential Diagnosis

1. Myocardial ischemia or infarction
2. Cocaine-induced myocardial ischemia
3. GERD
4. Aortic dissection
5. Pericarditis
6. Pneumothorax
7. Pulmonary embolism
8. Costochondritis

### Diagnostic Workup

1. ECG
2. Cardiac enzymes (CPK, CPK-MB, troponin)
3. CXR
4. Transthoracic echocardiogram
5. Cardiac catheterization
6. Transesophageal echocardiogram
7. CT—chest with IV contrast
8. Upper endoscopy
9. Cholesterol panel

# CASE DISCUSSION

## Differential Diagnosis

- **Myocardial ischemia or infarction:** The patient has multiple cardiac risk factors (including smoking, hypertension, and hyperlipidemia), and his symptoms are classic for cardiac ischemia.
- **Cocaine-induced:** Cocaine can predispose to premature atherosclerosis or can induce myocardial ischemia and infarction by causing coronary artery vasoconstriction or by increasing myocardial energy requirements.
- **GERD:** Severe chest pain is atypical but not uncommon for GERD and may worsen with recumbency overnight. Other atypical symptoms may include chronic cough, wheezing, or dysphagia. The classic symptom of GERD is heartburn, which may be exacerbated by meals.
- **Aortic dissection:** With the sudden onset of severe chest pain, aortic dissection should be suspected given the high potential for death if missed (and the potential for harm if mistaken for acute MI and treated with thrombolytic therapy). However, the patient's pain is not the classic sudden tearing chest pain that radiates to the back. In addition, his peripheral pulses and blood pressures are not diminished or unequal, and there is no aortic regurgitant murmur (although physical exam findings have poor sensitivity and specificity to diagnose aortic dissection).
- **Pericarditis:** The absence of pain that changes with position or respiration and the absence of a pericardial friction rub make pericarditis less likely.
- **Pneumothorax:** This diagnosis should be entertained in a patient with acute chest pain and difficulty breathing, but it is less likely in this case given that breath sounds are symmetric.
- **Pulmonary embolism:** As above, this is on the differential for acute chest pain and difficulty breathing, but this patient has no apparent risk factors for pulmonary embolism.
- **Costochondritis (or other musculoskeletal chest pain):** This is more typically associated with pain on palpation or pleuritic pain.

## Diagnostic Workup

- **ECG:** Acute myocardial ischemia, infarction, and pericarditis have characteristic changes on ECG.
- **Cardiac enzymes (CPK, CPK-MB, troponin):** Specific tests for myocardial tissue necrosis that can turn positive as early as 4–6 hours after onset of pain.
- **CXR:** A widened mediastinum suggests aortic dissection and can also diagnose other causes of chest pain, including pneumothorax and pneumonia.
- **Transthoracic echocardiogram (TTE):** Can demonstrate segmental wall motion abnormalities in suspected acute MIs (infarction is unlikely in the absence of wall motion abnormalities).
- **Cardiac catheterization:** Can diagnose and treat coronary artery disease.
- **Transesophageal echocardiogram (TEE):** Highly specific and sensitive for aortic dissection, and can be done rapidly at the bedside.
- **CT–chest with IV contrast:** Another rapidly available diagnostic study that can rule out aortic dissection or pulmonary embolism.
- **Upper endoscopy:** Can be used to document tissue damage characteristic of GERD. However, it can be normal in up to one-half of symptomatic patients; esophageal probe (pH and manometry measurements) together with endoscopic visualization constitutes an effective diagnostic technique.
- **Cholesterol panel:** Can identify a critical risk factor for cardiovascular disease.

## DOORWAY INFORMATION

### Opening Scenario

The mother of Josh White, a seven-month-old male child, comes to the office complaining that her child has a fever.

### Examinee Tasks

1. Take a focused history.
2. Explain your clinical impression and workup plan to the mother.
3. Write the patient note after leaving the room.

### Checklist/SP Sheet

PATIENT DESCRIPTION

The patient's mother offers the history; she is a fair historian.

NOTES FOR THE SP

Show concern regarding your child's situation.

CHALLENGING QUESTIONS TO ASK

- "Is my child going to be okay?"
- "Do you think I need to bring my child to the hospital?"

SAMPLE EXAMINEE RESPONSE

"Well, I will need to examine your child first. Although I suspect that he has a viral infection, I still need to make sure that he does not have anything else."

### Examinee Checklist

ENTRANCE:

☐ Examinee knocked on the door before entering.
☐ Examinee introduced self by name.
☐ Examinee identified his/her role or position.
☐ Examinee correctly used patient's name.
☐ Examinee made eye contact with the SP.

HISTORY:

☐ Examinee showed compassion for your child's illness.

| ☑ **Question** | **Patient Response** |
| --- | --- |
| ☐ Chief complaint | My child has a fever. |
| ☐ Onset | Yesterday. |
| ☐ Temperature | I measured it, and it was 101. |
| ☐ Runny nose | Yes. |
| ☐ Ear pulling/ear discharge | No. |
| ☐ Cough | No. |
| ☐ Shortness of breath | I think so; he is breathing quickly and using stomach muscles to breathe. |
| ☐ Difficulty swallowing | I don't know, but he hasn't eaten anything since yesterday and is refusing to drink from his bottle or my breast. |
| ☐ Rash | No. |
| ☐ Nausea/vomiting | No. |
| ☐ Change in bowel habits or in stool color or consistency | No. |
| ☐ Change in urinary habits or urine smell or color, making normal number of wet diapers | No. |
| ☐ Shaking (seizures) | No. |
| ☐ How has the baby looked (lethargic, irritated, playful, etc.)? | He has looked tired and irritated since yesterday. |
| ☐ Appetite changes | He is not eating anything at all. |
| ☐ Ill contacts | His three-year-old brother had an upper respiratory tract infection one week ago, and he is fine now. |
| ☐ Day care center | Yes. |
| ☐ Ill contacts in day care center | I don't know. |
| ☐ Vaccinations | Up to date. |
| ☐ Last checkup | Two weeks ago, and everything was perfect with him. |
| ☐ Birth history | It was a 40-week vaginal delivery with no complications. |
| ☐ Child weight, height, and language development | Normal. |
| ☐ Eating habits | I am breast-feeding him, and I give him all the vitamins that his pediatrician prescribes. He has refused my breast since yesterday. He also gets baby food three times a day. |
| ☐ Sleeping habits | Last night he did not sleep well and cried when I laid him down. |
| ☐ Current medications | Tylenol. |
| ☐ Past medical history | Jaundice in the first week of life. |

| ✓ | Question | Patient Response |
|---|----------|------------------|
| ☐ | Past surgical history | None. |
| ☐ | Drug allergies | No. |

## Physical Examination:

None.

## Closure:

☐ Examinee discussed initial diagnostic impressions.

☐ Examinee discussed initial management plans:

    ☐ Follow-up tests.

☐ Examinee asked if the patient has any other questions or concerns.

**USMLE**
STEP 2 CS

# PATIENT NOTE

**History**

**Physical Examination**

**Differential Diagnosis**

1.
2.
3.
4.
5.

**Diagnostic Workup**

1.
2.
3.
4.
5.

## History

**HPI:** *The source of information is the patient's mother. The mother of a 7-month-old M c/o her child having a fever of 101°F since yesterday. For the past day, the child has been tired, irritated, and breathing rapidly. The mother notes that yesterday the child also had a runny nose, did not sleep well, and refused her breast and baby food. There is a history of ill contact with his 3-year-old brother, who had a URI 1 week ago but is recovered now. The child goes to a day care center. The mother denies cough, ear pulling, ear discharge, or rash.*
**ROS:** *Negative except as above.*
**Allergies:** *NKDA.*
**Medications:** *Tylenol.*
**PMH:** *Jaundice in the first week of life.*
**Birth history:** *40-week vaginal delivery with no complications.*
**Dietary history:** *Breast-feeding and supplemental vitamins.*
**Immunization history:** *UTD.*
**Developmental history:** *Last checkup was 2 weeks ago and showed normal weight, height, hearing/vision, and developmental milestones.*

## Physical Examination

*None.*

## Differential Diagnosis

1. Viral URI
2. Pneumonia
3. Meningitis
4. UTI
5. Otitis media
6. Gastroenteritis
7. Occult bacteremia

## Diagnostic Workup

1. Pneumatic otoscopy
2. Tympanometry
3. CBC with differential, blood culture, UA and urine culture
4. LP—CSF analysis
5. CT—head
6. CXR
7. Bronchoscopy
8. Serum antibody titers
9. U/S—renal
10. Voiding cystourethrogram

## CASE DISCUSSION

### Differential Diagnosis

- **Viral URI:** Possible clues suggesting this diagnosis as the source of fever include rhinorrhea and recent exposure to a sibling with URI. It is probably viral, self-limited, and benign, but lower respiratory tract infection must first be ruled out in light of the child's apparent dyspnea and tachypnea.
- **Pneumonia:** Fever, rhinorrhea, tachypnea, and dyspnea support this diagnosis, although cough is not present. The physical exam may find retractions, nasal flaring, grunting, dullness on chest percussion, and rales.
- **Meningitis:** Findings are often subtle and nonspecific and may be limited to fever, irritability, and poor feeding, as seen in this case. The physical exam may reveal a bulging fontanelle; meningeal signs may not be obvious in infants (nuchal rigidity and focal neurologic signs are more commonly seen in older children).
- **UTI:** Infants with UTI may not have symptoms referable to the urinary tract. Those who do may have dribbling or colic before and during voiding. Patients with high fever and CVA tenderness are presumed to have pyelonephritis until proven otherwise.
- **Otitis media:** Otalgia and ear drainage can suggest this diagnosis in an ill, febrile child but are often not present (as in this case). The physical exam is key and may reveal a hyperemic, bulging TM; loss of TM landmarks; and decreased TM mobility.
- **Gastroenteritis:** This patient has fever but no GI symptoms. Viral infection typically causes vomiting and/or watery diarrhea, whereas bacterial infection may cause fever, tenesmus, bloody diarrhea, and severe abdominal pain.
- **Occult bacteremia:** This is an important consideration for children with high fever (> 102°F/38.9°C) and no obvious source. There is a relatively high proportion of children with no identifiable fever source who will have a positive blood culture, which can progress to sepsis if untreated. An extensive workup (see below) is not necessarily indicated in this case, as fever is < 102°F (38.9°C).

### Diagnostic Workup

- **Pneumatic otoscopy:** Key to look for the decreased TM mobility seen in otitis media.
- **Tympanometry:** Useful in infants > 6 months of age; confirms abnormal TM mobility in otitis media.
- **CBC with differential, blood culture, UA and urine culture:** Constitutes the "septic" or occult bacteremia workup in children with unexplained high fever. Notably, a WBC count > 15,000/μL is suggestive of occult bacteremia. UTI may be occult and must be investigated.
- **LP—CSF analysis:** Should be performed if there is **any** concern for meningitis. CSF analysis includes cell count and differential, glucose, protein, Gram stain, culture, latex agglutination for common bacterial antigens, and occasionally PCR for specific viruses.
- **CT—head:** Used mainly to rule out brain abscess or hemorrhage.
- **CXR:** To diagnose pneumonia.
- **Bronchoscopy:** A diagnostic aid in severe or refractory pneumonia cases.
- **Serum antibody titers:** To identify causative viruses in pediatric infections (not commonly used).
- **U/S—renal:** To look for anatomic anomalies that predispose to UTI.
- **Voiding cystourethrogram:** To look for vesicoureteral reflux in UTI.

### Opening Scenario

The mother of Maria Sterling, an 18-month-old female child, comes to the office complaining that her child has a fever.

### Examinee Tasks

1. Take a focused history.
2. Explain your clinical impression and workup plan to the mother.
3. Write the patient note after leaving the room.

### Checklist/SP Sheet

#### PATIENT DESCRIPTION

The patient's mother offers the history; the child is at home.

#### NOTES FOR THE SP

Show concern regarding your child's situation.

#### CHALLENGING QUESTIONS TO ASK

- "Do you think that I did the right thing by coming here and telling you about my child's fever?"
- "Is my child going to be okay?"

#### SAMPLE EXAMINEE RESPONSE

"You absolutely did the right thing. Maria may have an infection that needs antibiotics; we need to examine her here in the office and then decide whether she needs any more testing or treatment."

### Examinee Checklist

#### ENTRANCE:

- ☐ Examinee knocked on the door before entering.
- ☐ Examinee introduced self by name.
- ☐ Examinee identified his/her role or position.
- ☐ Examinee correctly used patient's name.
- ☐ Examinee made eye contact with the SP.

#### HISTORY:

- ☐ Examinee showed compassion for your child's illness.

| ☑ | Question | Patient Response |
|---|----------|------------------|
| ☐ | Chief complaint | My child has a fever. |
| ☐ | Onset | Two days ago. |
| ☐ | Temperature | I measured it, and it was 101°F rectally. |
| ☐ | Runny nose | No. |
| ☐ | Ear pulling/discharge | Yes, she has been pulling at her right ear for two days. |
| ☐ | Cough | No. |
| ☐ | Shortness of breath | No. |
| ☐ | Difficulty swallowing | She feels pain while she is eating her food. |
| ☐ | Rash | Yes, she has some sort of rash on her face and chest. |
| ☐ | Description of the rash | Tiny red dots, some slightly elevated over the chest, back, belly, and face. There is no rash on her arms or legs. |
| ☐ | Onset of rash and progression | It started two days ago on her face and then spread to her chest, back, and belly. |
| ☐ | Nausea/vomiting | No. |
| ☐ | Change in bowel habits or in stool color or consistency | No. |
| ☐ | Change in urinary habits or urine smell or color | No. |
| ☐ | Shaking (seizures) | No. |
| ☐ | How has the child looked (lethargic, irritated, playful, etc.)? | She looks tired. She is not playing with her toys today and is not watching TV the way she usually does. |
| ☐ | Appetite changes | She is not eating as usual but is drinking milk. |
| ☐ | Ill contacts | No. |
| ☐ | Day care center | Yes. |
| ☐ | Ill contacts in day care center | I don't know. |
| ☐ | Vaccinations | Up to date. |
| ☐ | Last checkup | One month ago, and everything was normal. |
| ☐ | Birth history | It was a 40-week vaginal delivery with no complications. |
| ☐ | Child weight, height, and language development | Normal. |
| ☐ | Eating habits | Whole milk and solid food; I did not breast-feed my child. |
| ☐ | Sleeping habits | She has not slept well for two days. |
| ☐ | Hearing problems | No. |
| ☐ | Vision problems | No. |
| ☐ | Current medications | Tylenol. |

| ✓ | Question | Patient Response |
|---|----------|------------------|
| ☐ | Past medical history | Three months ago she had an ear infection that was treated successfully with amoxicillin. |
| ☐ | Past surgical history | None. |
| ☐ | Drug allergies | No. |

## Physical Examination:

None.

## Closure:

☐ Examinee discussed initial diagnostic impressions.
☐ Examinee discussed initial management plans:
    ☐ Follow-up tests.
☐ Examinee asked if the patient has any other questions or concerns.

# PATIENT NOTE

**History**

**Physical Examination**

| Differential Diagnosis | Diagnostic Workup |
|---|---|
| 1. | 1. |
| 2. | 2. |
| 3. | 3. |
| 4. | 4. |
| 5. | 5. |

## History

**HPI:** *The source of information is the patient's mother. The mother of an 18-month-old F c/o her child having a fever for 2 days. She notes that the child is tired and is not playing with her toys or watching TV as she usually does. The mother recalls that her child has been pulling at her right ear and having difficulty swallowing and sleeping for the past 2 days. The child also developed a maculopapular facial rash that then spread over the chest, back, and abdomen. There is no rash on her arms or legs. The child also has loss of appetite. She goes to a day care center, but there is no known history of ill contact. The mother denies cough or ear discharge.*
**ROS:** *Negative except as above.*
**Allergies:** *NKDA.*
**Medications:** *Tylenol.*
**PMH:** *Otitis media 3 months ago, treated with amoxicillin.*
**Birth history:** *40-week vaginal delivery with no complications.*
**Dietary history:** *Formula milk and solid food. She was not breast-fed.*
**Immunization history:** *UTD.*
**Developmental history:** *Last checkup was 1 month ago and showed normal weight, height, hearing, vision, and developmental milestones.*

## Physical Examination

*None.*

## Differential Diagnosis

1. Otitis media
2. Meningococcal meningitis
3. Scarlet fever
4. Fifth disease or other viral exanthem
5. Varicella

## Diagnostic Workup

1. Pneumatic otoscopy
2. Tympanometry
3. LP—CSF analysis
4. Platelets, PT/PTT, D-dimer, fibrin split products, fibrinogen
5. CBC with differential, blood culture, UA and urine culture
6. Throat culture
7. Parvovirus B19 IgM antibody
8. Skin lesion scrapings
9. Varicella antibody titer

# CASE DISCUSSION

## Differential Diagnosis

- **Otitis media:** Fever and otalgia suggest this diagnosis but are present in < 50% of patients. Physical exam is key and may reveal a hyperemic, bulging TM; loss of TM landmarks; and decreased TM mobility.
- **Meningococcal meningitis:** Fever, lethargy, and a possible petechial rash are worrisome for meningococcemia. Patients may also have headache, vomiting, photophobia, neck stiffness, and seizures. This is a severe, rapidly progressive, and sometimes fatal infection; the patient would appear very ill.
- **Scarlet fever:** This patient has fever, difficulty swallowing (i.e., possible pharyngitis), and a rash that started on her face and spread to the trunk. However, the description does not allow one to ascertain whether or not the rash consists of a diffuse erythema with punctate elevations resembling sandpaper that spares the area around the mouth. Also, scarlet fever is more common in school-age children.
- **Fifth disease or other viral exanthem:** In children, viruses commonly present with low-grade fever and rash. In general, viral exanthems are quite nonspecific in their appearance and are usually maculopapular and diffuse. Parvovirus B19 infection, or fifth disease, usually presents as intense, red facial flushing ("slapped cheek" appearance) that then spreads over the trunk and becomes more diffuse. Rubeola classically presents as 2–5 days of high fever followed by a diffuse rash. However, almost any virus can be accompanied by rash in the pediatric patient, and it is not always necessary to ascertain which virus is causing the illness. If the illness is prolonged or particularly troublesome, antibody titers can be ordered to determine the exact etiology of the illness.
- **Varicella:** Fever and rash, along with day care attendance, could be consistent with this infection. However, in varicella the lesions are present in various stages of development at any given time (i.e., red macules, vesicles, pustules, crusting), and the rash is intensely pruritic. The incidence of varicella has declined since vaccination began in the 1990s.

## Diagnostic Workup

- **Pneumatic otoscopy:** Key to look for the decreased TM mobility seen in otitis media.
- **Tympanometry:** Useful in infants > 6 months of age; confirms abnormal TM mobility in otitis media.
- **LP–CSF analysis:** Should be performed if there is **any** concern for meningitis. CSF analysis includes cell count and differential, glucose, protein, Gram stain, culture, latex agglutination for common bacterial antigens, and occasionally PCR for specific viruses.
- **Platelets, PT/PTT, D-dimer, fibrin split products, fibrinogen:** Evidence of DIC is often seen in meningococcemia.
- **CBC with differential, blood culture, UA and urine culture:** To isolate *Neisseria meningitidis* and to screen for occult bacteremia or UTI.
- **Throat culture:** To isolate *Streptococcus pyogenes* (causes scarlet fever). The rash is pathognomonic for this diagnosis.
- **Parvovirus B19 IgM antibody:** The best marker of acute or recent infection in suspected fifth disease.
- **Skin lesion scrapings:** Varicella antigens are identified by PCR or direct immunofluorescence (DFA) of skin lesions. Also, a Tzanck smear may show multinucleated giant cells in varicella infection.
- **Varicella antibody titer:** May be useful in uncertain cases (look for a fourfold rise in antibody titer following acute infection).

### Opening Scenario

Eric Glenn, a 26-year-old male, comes to the office complaining of cough.

### Vital Signs

**BP:** 120/80 mmHg
**Temp:** 99.5°F (37.5°C)
**RR:** 15/minute
**HR:** 75/minute, regular

### Examinee Tasks

1. Take a focused history.
2. Perform a focused physical exam (do not perform rectal, genitourinary, or female breast exam).
3. Explain your clinical impression and workup plan to the patient.
4. Write the patient note after leaving the room.

### Checklist/SP Sheet

PATIENT DESCRIPTION

Patient is a 26 yo M.

NOTES FOR THE SP

- Cough as the examinee enters the room.
- Continue coughing every 3–4 minutes during the encounter.
- Chest auscultation: When asked to take a breath while the examinee is listening to your right chest, pretend to inhale by moving your shoulders up, but do not actually breathe in.
- Chest palpation: When the examinee palpates your right chest and asks you to say "99," turn your face to the right side, and say it in a coarse, deep voice.
- If asked about sputum, ask the examinee, "What does 'sputum' mean?"
- During the encounter, pretend to have a severe attack of coughing. Note whether the examinee offers you a glass of water or a tissue.

CHALLENGING QUESTIONS TO ASK

"Do I need antibiotics to get better?"

SAMPLE EXAMINEE RESPONSE

"Maybe. Antibiotics don't help in bronchitis, but they will help if we find pneumonia."

## Examinee Checklist

### ENTRANCE:

- ☐ Examinee knocked on the door before entering.
- ☐ Examinee introduced self by name.
- ☐ Examinee identified his/her role or position.
- ☐ Examinee correctly used patient's name.
- ☐ Examinee made eye contact with the SP.

### HISTORY:

- ☐ Examinee showed compassion for your illness.
- ☐ Examinee offered you a glass of water or a tissue during your severe bout of coughing.

| ☑ Question | Patient Response |
|---|---|
| ☐ Chief complaint | Cough. |
| ☐ Onset | One week ago. |
| ☐ Preceding symptoms/events | Runny nose, fever, sore throat two weeks ago for one week, which then resolved. |
| ☐ Fever/chills | Mild fever, but I didn't take my temperature; no chills. |
| ☐ Sputum production | Small amounts of white mucus. |
| ☐ Blood in sputum | No. |
| ☐ Chest pain | Yes, I feel a sharp pain when I cough or take a deep breath. |
| ☐ Location | Right chest. |
| ☐ Quality | It is like a knife. I can't take a deep breath. |
| ☐ Alleviating/exacerbating factors | It increases when I take a deep breath and when I cough. I feel better when I sleep on my right side. |
| ☐ Radiation of pain | No. |
| ☐ Severity on a scale | 8/10. |
| ☐ Night sweats | No. |
| ☐ Exposure to TB | None. |
| ☐ Pet, animal exposure | None. |
| ☐ Recent travel | None. |
| ☐ Last PPD | Never had it. |
| ☐ Associated symptoms (shortness of breath, wheezing, abdominal pain, nausea/vomiting, diarrhea/constipation) | None. |
| ☐ Weight/appetite changes | No. |
| ☐ Current medications | Tylenol. |

| ☑ Question | Patient Response |
|---|---|
| ☐ Past medical history | I had gonorrhea two years ago and was cured after a course of antibiotics. |
| ☐ Past surgical history | None. |
| ☐ Family history | My father and mother are alive and in good health. |
| ☐ Occupation | Pizza delivery boy. |
| ☐ Alcohol use | I drink a lot on the weekends. I never count. |
| ☐ Illicit drug use | Never. |
| ☐ Tobacco | Yes, I smoke one pack a day. I started when I was 15 years old. |
| ☐ Sexual activity | Well, I've had many girlfriends. Every Saturday night, I pick up a new girl from the nightclub. |
| ☐ Use of condoms | Nope, I don't enjoy it with a condom. |
| ☐ Drug allergies | No. |

## Physical Examination:

☐ Examinee washed his/her hands.
☐ Examinee asked permission to start the exam.
☐ Examinee used respectful draping.
☐ Examinee did not repeat painful maneuvers.

| ☑ Exam Component | Maneuver |
|---|---|
| ☐ Head and neck exam | Examined mouth, throat, lymph nodes |
| ☐ CV exam | Auscultation, palpation |
| ☐ Pulmonary exam | Auscultation, palpation, percussion |
| ☐ Extremities | Inspection |

## Closure:

☐ Examinee discussed initial diagnostic impressions.
☐ Examinee discussed initial management plans:
    ☐ Follow-up tests.
    ☐ Discussed safe sex practices.
    ☐ Recommended HIV testing (and discussed consent).
☐ Examinee asked if the patient has any other questions or concerns.

**USMLE STEP 2 CS** PATIENT NOTE

**History**

**Physical Examination**

**Differential Diagnosis**

1.

2.

3.

4.

5.

**Diagnostic Workup**

1.

2.

3.

4.

5.

## History

**HPI:** *26 yo M c/o cough for 1 week. Two weeks ago the patient had a fever, runny nose, and sore throat. These symptoms resolved and were followed by a cough that has persisted. The cough is productive of small amounts of white mucus with no blood. The patient also notes a sharp, stabbing 8/10 pain in the right chest that occurs with and is exacerbated by coughing and deep inspiration. He has a mild fever but denies chills, night sweats, shortness of breath, or wheezing. The patient has not traveled recently and denies exposure to TB. There are no weight or appetite changes.*
**ROS:** *Negative except as above.*
**Allergies:** *NKDA.*
**Medications:** *Tylenol.*
**PMH:** *Gonorrhea 2 years ago, treated with antibiotics.*
**SH:** *One PPD since age 15; drinks heavily on weekends. Unprotected sex with multiple female partners.*
**FH:** *Noncontributory.*

## Physical Examination

*Patient is in no acute distress.*
**VS:** *WNL.*
**HEENT:** *Nose, mouth, and pharynx WNL.*
**Neck:** *No JVD, no lymphadenopathy.*
**Chest:** *Increase in tactile fremitus and decrease in breath sounds on the right side. No rhonchi, rales, or wheezing.*
**Heart:** *Apical impulse not displaced; RRR; normal S1/S2; no murmurs, rubs, or gallops.*
**Extremities:** *No cyanosis or edema.*

## Differential Diagnosis

1. URI-associated ("postinfectious") cough
2. Acute bronchitis
3. Pneumonia
4. Pleurodynia
5. Aspiration

## Diagnostic Workup

1. CXR
2. CBC
3. Sputum Gram stain and culture
4. Urine *Legionella* antigen, serum *Mycoplasma* PCR, cold agglutinin measurement
5. Bronchoscopy with bronchoalveolar lavage
6. Pulse oximetry or ABG
7. HIV antibody

# CASE DISCUSSION

## Differential Diagnosis

This young man's acute productive cough and pleuritic pain are likely caused by viral respiratory infection or pneumonia. Rarely, severe coughing can lead to a rib fracture, which in turn can cause severe pleuritis.

- **URI-associated cough:** Acute cough frequently follows URI ("**postinfectious**") and can commonly persist for 1–2 weeks (or up to 6–8 weeks in patients with underlying asthma). URIs range from rhinosinusitis to acute bronchitis.
- **Acute bronchitis:** Cough can also accompany acute URI.
- **Pneumonia:** Pleuritic pain may signal lower respiratory tract infection. This diagnosis is often confirmed by characteristic chest exam findings, which may be difficult to elicit in an otherwise healthy SP. Increased tactile fremitus suggests airspace consolidation, but there are no bronchial breath sounds or rales to help suggest a focal pneumonia. Also, the absence of dyspnea argues against this diagnosis.
- **Pleurodynia:** An uncommon acute illness usually caused by one of the coxsackieviruses. It occurs in summer and early fall and presents with acute severe paroxysmal pain of the thorax or abdomen that worsens with cough or breathing. Most patients recover within three days to one week.
- **Other etiologies:** Other causes of acute cough include aspiration (alcoholics, elderly, and neurologically impaired are at risk), pulmonary embolism (extremely rare in a young patient with no risk factors), and pulmonary edema (signs and symptoms of heart failure would be present). Given the patient's history of STD, he should be screened for HIV infection. Notably, there is no evidence of immunosuppression on exam (e.g., no thrush), and in PCP pneumonia cough is usually nonproductive and accompanied by dyspnea.

## Diagnostic Workup

- **CXR:** To help diagnose pneumonia (i.e., to see infiltrates, effusion), although a normal film does not necessarily rule it out.
- **CBC:** In acute infection, can reveal leukopenia or leukocytosis.
- **Sputum Gram stain and culture:** Often low yield (due to contamination by oral flora and often discordant results between Gram stain and culture in pneumococcal pneumonia), but may help identify a microbiologic diagnosis in pneumonia.
- **Urine *Legionella* antigen, serum *Mycoplasma* PCR, cold agglutinin measurement:** To help diagnose specific causes of atypical pneumonia. Usually **not** useful in the initial evaluation of patients with community-acquired pneumonia.
- **Bronchoscopy with bronchoalveolar lavage:** An invasive test that is rarely necessary to diagnose community-acquired pneumonia, but a gold standard that is often used early when PCP infection is suspected.
- **Pulse oximetry or ABG:** May help determine the need for hospitalization.
- **HIV antibody:** Should be offered to all patients with risk factors for this infection.

## Opening Scenario

Marilyn McLean, a 54-year-old female, comes to the office complaining of persistent cough.

## Vital Signs

**BP:** 120/80 mmHg
**Temp:** 99.5°F (37.5°C)
**RR:** 15/minute
**HR:** 75/minute, regular.

## Examinee Tasks

1. Take a focused history.
2. Perform a focused physical exam (do not perform rectal, genitourinary, or female breast exam).
3. Explain your clinical impression and workup plan to the patient.
4. Write the patient note after leaving the room.

## Checklist/SP Sheet

PATIENT DESCRIPTION

Patient is a 54 yo F.

NOTES FOR THE SP

- Cough as the examinee enters the room.
- Continue coughing every 3–4 minutes during the encounter.
- Hold a tissue in your hand, with red staining to simulate blood. Don't show it to the examinee unless he/she asks you.
- If asked about sputum, ask the examinee, "What does 'sputum' mean?"
- During the encounter, pretend to have a severe attack of coughing. Note whether the examinee offers you a glass of water or a tissue.

CHALLENGING QUESTIONS TO ASK

"Will I get better if I stop smoking?"

SAMPLE EXAMINEE RESPONSE

"Well, we still have to sort out exactly what's making you sick. Stopping smoking should help your chronic cough, and over the long term it will significantly decrease your cancer risk."

## Examinee Checklist

ENTRANCE:

☐ Examinee knocked on the door before entering.
☐ Examinee introduced self by name.

☐ Examinee identified his/her role or position.

☐ Examinee correctly used patient's name.

☐ Examinee made eye contact with the SP.

## HISTORY:

☐ Examinee showed compassion for your illness.

☐ Examinee offered you a glass of water or a tissue during your severe bout of coughing.

| ☑ Question | Patient Response |
|---|---|
| ☐ Chief complaint | Persistent cough. |
| ☐ Onset | I've had a cough for years, especially in the morning. This past month, the cough has gotten worse, and it is really annoying me. |
| ☐ Changes of the cough during the day | No. |
| ☐ Progression of the cough during the last month | It is getting worse. |
| ☐ Do you cough at night? | Yes, sometimes I can't sleep because of it. |
| ☐ Alleviating/exacerbating factors | Nothing. |
| ☐ Sputum production<br>☐ Amount<br>☐ Color<br>☐ Odor<br>☐ Blood<br>☐ Amount of blood | Yes.<br>Two teaspoonfuls, stable.<br>Yellowish mucus.<br>None.<br>Yes, recently.<br>Streaks. |
| ☐ Preceding symptoms/events | None. |
| ☐ Fever/chills | Mild, especially at night. I didn't take my temperature. I have had no chills. |
| ☐ Night sweats | Yes. |
| ☐ Chest pain | No. |
| ☐ Shortness of breath | Yes, when I walk up the stairs. |
| ☐ Exposure to TB | Yes, I work in a nursing home, and several of our residents are under treatment for TB. |
| ☐ Recent travel | None. |
| ☐ Last PPD | Last year, before I started working in the nursing home. It was negative. |
| ☐ Associated symptoms (wheezing, abdominal pain, nausea/vomiting, diarrhea/constipation) | None. |
| ☐ Appetite changes | Yes, I don't have an appetite. |

| ☑ Question | Patient Response |
|---|---|
| ☐ Weight changes | Yes, I lost six pounds in the last two months. |
| ☐ Fatigue<br>☐ Since when | Yes, I don't have the energy that I had before.<br>Two months ago. |
| ☐ Current medications | Cough syrup "over the counter," multivitamins, albuterol inhaler. |
| ☐ Past medical history | Chronic bronchitis. |
| ☐ Past surgical history | Tonsillectomy and adenoidectomy, age 11. |
| ☐ Family history | My father died of old age. My mother is alive and has Alzheimer's. |
| ☐ Occupation | Nurse. |
| ☐ Alcohol use | None. |
| ☐ Illicit drug use | Never. |
| ☐ Tobacco | No, I stopped smoking two weeks ago. |
| ☐ Duration | I smoked for the past 35 years. |
| ☐ Amount | One to two packs a day. |
| ☐ Sexual activity | With my husband. |
| ☐ Drug allergies | No. |

## Physical Examination:

☐ Examinee washed his/her hands.

☐ Examinee asked permission to start the exam.

☐ Examinee used respectful draping.

☐ Examinee did not repeat painful maneuvers.

| ☑ Exam Component | Maneuver |
|---|---|
| ☐ Head and neck exam | Inspected mouth, throat, lymph nodes |
| ☐ CV exam | Auscultation |
| ☐ Pulmonary exam | Auscultation, palpation, percussion |
| ☐ Abdominal exam | Auscultation, palpation |
| ☐ Extremities | Inspection |

## Closure:

☐ Examinee discussed initial diagnostic impressions.

☐ Examinee discussed initial management plans.

☐ Examinee asked if the patient has any other questions or concerns.

**USMLE**
STEP 2 CS

# PATIENT NOTE

**History**

**Physical Examination**

**Differential Diagnosis**

1.
2.
3.
4.
5.

**Diagnostic Workup**

1.
2.
3.
4.
5.

## History

**HPI:** *54 yo F with PMH of chronic bronchitis c/o worsening cough over the last month. The cough is productive of 2 teaspoonfuls of yellowish mucus, with occasional streaks of blood. Patient notes dyspnea on exertion. She also has fever and sweats at night. No chest pain or wheezing. No chills. The patient reports fatigue, decreased appetite, and a weight loss of 6 pounds during the last 2 months. No recent travel. Exposed to patients with TB in the nursing home, where she works as a nurse. Her last PPD test was last year and was negative.*
**ROS:** *Negative except as above.*
**Allergies:** *NKDA.*
**Medications:** *OTC cough syrup, multivitamins, albuterol inhaler.*
**PMH:** *Per HPI.*
**PSH:** *Tonsillectomy and adenoidectomy, age 11.*
**SH:** *One to two PPD for 35 years; stopped 2 weeks ago. No EtOH. Sexually active with husband only.*
**FH:** *Noncontributory.*

## Physical Examination

*Patient is in no acute distress.*
**VS:** *WNL.*
**HEENT:** *Mouth and pharynx WNL.*
**Neck:** *No JVD, no lymphadenopathy.*
**Chest:** *Clear breath sounds bilaterally; no rhonchi, rales, or wheezing; tactile fremitus normal.*
**Heart:** *Apical impulse not displaced; RRR; normal S1/S2; no murmurs, rubs, or gallops.*
**Abdomen:** *Soft, nontender, ⊕BS, no hepatosplenomegaly.*
**Extremities:** *No clubbing, cyanosis, or edema.*

## Differential Diagnosis

1. Pulmonary tuberculosis
2. Lung cancer
3. Lung abscess
4. Atypical pneumonia
5. Typical pneumonia
6. COPD exacerbation
7. Wegener's granulomatosis

## Diagnostic Workup

1. CBC
2. c-ANCA
3. Blood cultures
4. PPD
5. Sputum Gram stain, AFB smear, routine and mycobacterial sputum cultures, and cytology
6. CXR—PA and lateral
7. CT—chest
8. Bronchoscopy
9. Lung biopsy

# CASE DISCUSSION

## Differential Diagnosis

- **Pulmonary tuberculosis:** Clinical suspicion is high for this given the constitutional symptoms, hemoptysis, and recent exposure to active TB. The patient should be placed in respiratory isolation immediately.
- **Lung cancer:** As noted above, constitutional symptoms and hemoptysis in a long-time smoker are worrisome for cancer.
- **Lung abscess:** A lung abscess due to anaerobic bacteria is usually associated with a gradual onset of fatigue, fever, night sweats, cough producing a foul-smelling expectoration, and weight loss. Symptoms evolve over a period of weeks or months (the time course in this case favors abscess over uncomplicated pneumonia). Other bacterial causes of lung abscess typically present more acutely.
- **Atypical pneumonia:** Refers to infection by *Mycoplasma pneumoniae*, *Chlamydia pneumoniae*, and *Legionella* species. These can all present similarly with an insidious onset of fever, malaise, headache, myalgia, sore throat, hoarseness, chest pain, and nonproductive cough. Sputum may be blood-streaked. GI symptoms may be prominent in *Legionella* infection, and severe ear pain due to bullous myringitis may complicate up to 5% of *Mycoplasma* infections. The presence of weight loss and night sweats makes atypical pneumonia less likely in this case.
- **Typical pneumonia:** Classic bacterial pneumonia begins with abrupt onset of fever, chills, pleuritic chest pain, and productive cough. Remember that signs of pulmonary consolidation on physical exam are absent in up to two-thirds of documented cases. The more subacute time course seen here makes this diagnosis less likely.
- **COPD exacerbation:** This patient's baseline productive cough is due to COPD/chronic bronchitis secondary to tobacco exposure. Exacerbations of chronic bronchitis are more acute and involve increased sputum production and/or increased wheezing and dyspnea. Night sweats and weight loss are not typical features of this diagnosis.
- **Wegener's granulomatosis:** This rare small-vessel vasculitis usually develops over 4–12 months and classically involves the triad of upper respiratory tract, lower respiratory tract, and renal disease (which usually does not cause symptoms before the diagnosis is established). Constitutional symptoms are common. The absence of chronic upper respiratory complaints (e.g., sinusitis or nasal crusting) makes this diagnosis less likely.
- **Other etiologies:** Other common, benign causes of chronic cough include postnasal drip, GERD, asthma, and ACE inhibitors.

## Diagnostic Workup

- **CBC:** To identify leukocytosis in infection (nonspecific).
- **c-ANCA:** Highly specific (> 90%) and sensitive for active Wegener's granulomatosis.
- **Blood cultures:** May be useful in severe pneumonia to identify causative pathogenic bacteria.
- **PPD (tuberculin skin test):** Identifies individuals who have been infected with *Mycobacterium tuberculosis* but does not distinguish between active and latent infection.
- **Sputum Gram stain, AFB smear, routine and mycobacterial sputum cultures, and cytology:** To identify a causative agent of infection or to help detect malignancy.
- **CXR—PA and lateral:** To look for apical cavitary disease in TB reactivation, noncalcified nodules in lung cancer, a cavity with an air-fluid level in lung abscess, a patchy infiltrative pattern in atypical pneumonia, lobar consolidation in typical pneumonia, and infiltrates, nodules, masses, or cavities in Wegener's granulomatosis.
- **CT—chest:** May demonstrate lesions unseen on CXR, and aids in characterizing the size, shape, and composition of lung and mediastinal pathology. Can also guide diagnostic procedures (e.g., percutaneous transthoracic biopsies) and assist in staging.
- **Bronchoscopy:** Useful in diagnosing and staging lung cancer and in diagnosing infections.
- **Lung biopsy:** Can lead to definitive diagnosis. A range of techniques is used depending on the location of the tumor.

## Opening Scenario

Gail Abbott, a 52-year-old female, comes to the office complaining of yellow eyes and skin.

## Vital Signs

BP: 130/80 mmHg
Temp: 98.3°F (36.8°C)
RR: 15/minute
HR: 70/minute, regular

## Examinee Tasks

1. Take a focused history.
2. Perform a focused physical exam (do not perform rectal, genitourinary, or female breast exam).
3. Explain your clinical impression and workup plan to the patient.
4. Write the patient note after leaving the room.

## Checklist/SP Sheet

### PATIENT DESCRIPTION

Patient is a 52 yo F.

### NOTES FOR THE SP

- Sit up on the bed.
- Show signs of scratching.
- Exhibit RUQ tenderness on palpation.
- If ERCP, ultrasound, or MRI is mentioned, ask for an explanation.

### CHALLENGING QUESTIONS TO ASK

"My father had pancreatic cancer. Could I have it too?"

### SAMPLE EXAMINEE RESPONSE

"It's possible; that's why we always rule it out in patients with yellow eyes or skin. Your family history does put you at slightly increased risk, and we will keep that in mind."

## Examinee Checklist

### ENTRANCE:

☐ Examinee knocked on the door before entering.
☐ Examinee introduced self by name.
☐ Examinee identified his/her role or position.
☐ Examinee correctly used patient's name.
☐ Examinee made eye contact with the SP.

## HISTORY:

☐ Examinee showed compassion for your pain.

| ☑ Question | Patient Response |
|---|---|
| ☐ Chief complaint | Yellow eyes and skin. |
| ☐ Onset | Three weeks ago. |
| ☐ Color of stool | Light. |
| ☐ Color of urine | Dark. |
| ☐ Pruritus | I started itching two months ago; Benadryl used to help but not recently. |
| ☐ Abdominal pain | Sometimes. |
| ☐ Onset | It was around the same time that I noticed the change in the color of my eyes and skin. |
| ☐ Constant/intermittent | Well, I don't have the pain all the time. It comes and goes. |
| ☐ Frequency | At least once every day. |
| ☐ Progression | It is the same. |
| ☐ Severity on a scale | When I have the pain, it is 3/10, and then it may go down to 0. |
| ☐ Location | It is here (points to the RUQ). |
| ☐ Radiation | No. |
| ☐ Quality | Dull. |
| ☐ Alleviating factors | Tylenol. I take four pills every day just to make sure I do not feel the pain. |
| ☐ Exacerbating factors | None. |
| ☐ Relationship of food to pain | None. |
| ☐ Previous episodes of similar pain | No. |
| ☐ Nausea/vomiting | Sometimes I feel nauseated when I am in pain, but no vomiting. |
| ☑ Diarrhea/constipation | No. |
| ☐ Colonoscopy | Never. |
| ☐ Blood transfusion | Yes, when I had a C-section 20 years ago. |
| ☐ Fever, night sweats | No. |
| ☐ Fatigue | Yes, recently. |
| ☐ Weight changes | No. |
| ☐ Appetite changes | I have no appetite. |
| ☐ Joint pain | No. |
| ☐ Travel history | I went to Mexico for a brief vacation about two months ago. |

| ☑ *Question* | *Patient Response* |
|---|---|
| ☐ Immunization before travel | No. |
| ☐ Current medications | Tylenol, Synthroid. |
| ☐ Similar episodes | No. |
| ☐ Past medical history | Hypothyroidism. |
| ☐ Past surgical history | I had two C-sections at age 25 and 30 years and a tubal ligation at age 35. |
| ☐ Family history | My father died at 55 of pancreatic cancer. My mother is alive and healthy. |
| ☐ Occupation | I work in a travel agency. |
| ☐ Illicit drug use | No. |
| ☐ Tobacco | No. |
| ☐ Sexual activity | Yes, with my husband. |
| ☐ Drug allergies | Penicillin, causes rash. |
| ☐ How much alcohol do you drink?/Tell me about your use of alcohol | One or two glasses of wine every day for 30 years. |
| ☐ Have you ever felt a need to cut down on drinking? | No. |
| ☐ Have you ever felt annoyed by criticism of your drinking? | No. |
| ☐ Have you ever felt guilty about your drinking? | No, I heard that alcohol protects against heart disease. |
| ☐ Have you ever had a drink early in the morning ("eye opener") to steady your nerves or get rid of a hangover? | No. |
| ☐ Affecting job/relationships/legal problems | No. |

## Physical Examination:

- ☐ Examinee washed his/her hands.
- ☐ Examinee asked permission to start the exam.
- ☐ Examinee used respectful draping.
- ☐ Examinee did not repeat painful maneuvers.

| ☑ *Exam Component* | *Maneuver* |
|---|---|
| ☐ HEENT | Inspected sclerae, under tongue |
| ☐ CV exam | Auscultation |
| ☐ Pulmonary exam | Auscultation |
| ☐ Abdominal exam | Inspection, auscultation, palpation (including Murphy's sign), percussion |
| ☐ Extremities | Checked for asterixis, edema |
| ☐ Skin | Looked for spider nevi, cutaneous telangiectasias, palmar erythema |

## Closure:

☐ Examinee discussed initial diagnostic impressions.

☐ Examinee discussed initial management plans.

☐ Examinee asked if the patient has any other questions or concerns.

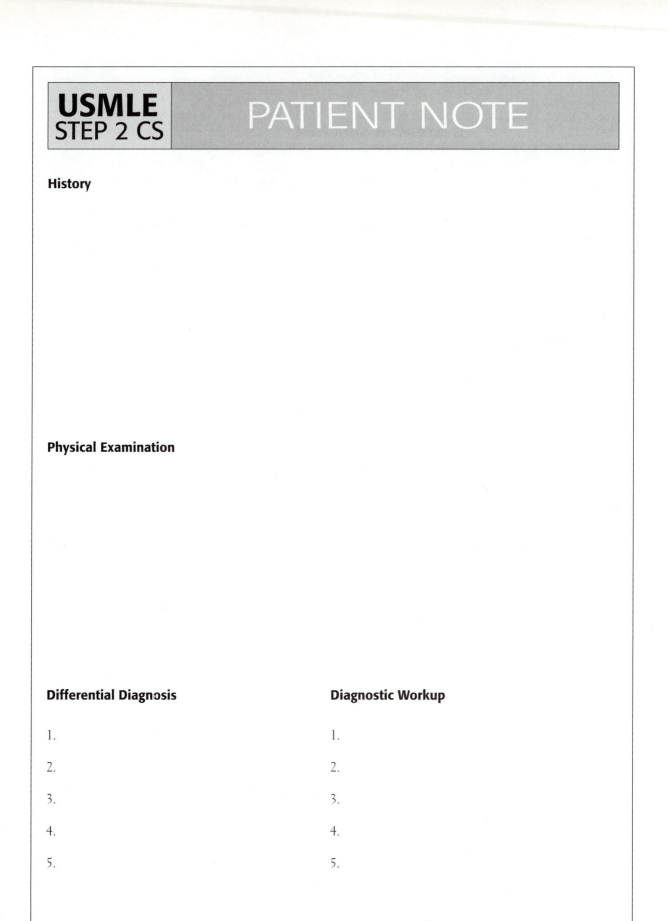

**USMLE**
STEP 2 CS

PATIENT NOTE

**History**

**Physical Examination**

**Differential Diagnosis**

1.

2.

3.

4.

5.

**Diagnostic Workup**

1.

2.

3.

4.

5.

## History

**HPI:** 52 yo F c/o yellow skin and eyes that started for the first time 3 weeks ago. Accompanied by light-colored stool and dark urine. Around the same time she also began having 3/10 RUQ pain that is dull and intermittent (at least daily), does not radiate, is unrelated to meals, and is relieved by Tylenol. There is associated anorexia, pruritus, and occasional nausea. She recently traveled to Mexico. No diarrhea, constipation, or weight loss. History of blood transfusion 20 years ago.

**ROS:** Negative except for fatigue.

**Allergies:** Penicillin, causes rash.

**Medications:** Tylenol, Synthroid.

**PMH:** Hypothyroidism.

**PSH:** Two C-sections, tubal ligation.

**SH:** No smoking, 1–2 glasses of wine/day for 30 years, CAGE 0/4, no illicit drugs. Sexually active with husband only.

**FH:** Father died of pancreatic cancer at age 55.

## Physical Examination

*Patient is in no acute distress.*

**VS:** WNL.

**HEENT:** Sclerae icteric.

**Chest:** Clear breath sounds bilaterally.

**Heart:** RRR; normal S1/S2; no murmurs, rubs, or gallops.

**Abdomen:** Soft, nondistended, C-section scar. Mild RUQ tenderness without rebound or guarding, ⊖Murphy's, ⊕BS, no organomegaly or masses. No evidence of ascites.

**Extremities:** No asterixis, no edema.

**Skin:** Jaundice, excoriations due to scratching, no spiders/telangiectasias/palmar erythema.

## Differential Diagnosis

1. Extrahepatic biliary obstruction:
   Pancreatic cancer
   Choledocholithiasis
   Cholangiocarcinoma
   Carcinoma of the ampulla
   Sphincter of Oddi dysfunction
2. Viral hepatitis
3. Acetaminophen liver toxicity
4. Alcoholic hepatitis
5. Primary biliary cirrhosis

## Diagnostic Workup

1. AST/ALT/bilirubin/alkaline phosphatase
2. CBC
3. PT/PTT
4. Viral hepatitis serologies
5. Acetaminophen level
6. U/S—abdomen
7. CT—abdomen
8. MRCP/ERCP

## CASE DISCUSSION

### Differential Diagnosis

Jaundice results from hyperbilirubinemia, the cause of which may be hepatic or nonhepatic. The presence of change in stool and urine color excludes unconjugated hyperbilirubinemia (e.g., that associated with hemolysis or Gilbert's syndrome). Thus, the predominantly conjugated hyperbilirubinemia suspected in this patient may be due to hepatocellular disease, drugs, sepsis, hereditary disorders such as Dubin-Johnson syndrome, or extrahepatic biliary obstruction. Cholangitis is ruled out by the absence of fever and chills associated with episodes of abdominal pain.

- **Extrahepatic biliary obstruction:** The patient's family history puts her at increased risk for **pancreatic cancer,** which classically presents with painless jaundice. However, her intermittent pain (suggesting intermittent biliary obstruction) narrows the differential to **choledocholithiasis** (stone in the common bile duct), **cholangiocarcinoma, carcinoma of the ampulla,** or **sphincter of Oddi dysfunction.**
- **Viral hepatitis:** The patient is at risk for hepatitis A (trip to Mexico) and chronic hepatitis C (remote blood transfusion). The intermittent nature of her RUQ pain makes acute hepatitis less likely.
- **Acetaminophen liver toxicity:** Suspect this in acute liver injury, and recognize that even moderate amounts of acetaminophen may overwhelm the metabolic capacity of a damaged liver (usually in alcoholics and in patients with chronic hepatitis or cirrhosis).
- **Alcoholic hepatitis:** The patient's symptoms are consistent with this diagnosis. Hepatomegaly is often present. Although she reports drinking only one or two glasses of wine daily, patients often underreport alcohol consumption.
- **Primary biliary cirrhosis.** This usually occurs in women aged 40–60, often with pruritus as a presenting symptom. However, jaundice is usually a late finding and is not associated with RUQ pain.

### Diagnostic Workup

- **AST/ALT/bilirubin/alkaline phosphatase:** Can help differentiate a hepatocellular process (primarily associated with increased AST and ALT) from a cholestatic process (primarily associated with increased bilirubin and alkaline phosphatase).
- **CBC:** A low platelet count is often seen in chronic liver disease, due to portal hypertension and subsequent splenomegaly.
- **PT/PTT:** A coagulopathy is often seen in advanced liver disease, due to synthetic dysfunction and subsequent clotting factor deficiencies.
- **Viral hepatitis serologies:** Check hepatitis A IgM antibody to document recent infection. Other screening tests include hepatitis B surface antigen and hepatitis C antibody.
- **Acetaminophen level:** To diagnose acetaminophen overdose.
- **U/S—abdomen:** Used to diagnose biliary obstruction, stones, or intrahepatic tumors.
- **CT—abdomen:** A CT scan provides information similar to that above but is more expensive.
- **MRCP/ERCP:** Can identify the cause, location, and extent of biliary obstruction. ERCP is invasive but has the advantage of being both a diagnostic and a therapeutic tool in many cases. MRCP is a noninvasive MRI-based diagnostic substitute.

## Opening Scenario

Virginia Black, a 65-year-old female, comes to the clinic complaining of forgetfulness and confusion.

## Vital Signs

**BP:** 135/90 mmHg
**Temp:** 98.0°F (36.7°C)
**RR:** 16/minute
**HR:** 76/minute, regular

## Examinee Tasks

1. Obtain a focused history.
2. Perform a focused physical exam (do not perform rectal, genitourinary, or female breast exam).
3. Explain your clinical impression and workup plan to the patient.
4. Write the patient note after leaving the room.

## Checklist/SP Sheet

### PATIENT DESCRIPTION

Patient is a 65 yo F, widowed with one daughter.

### NOTES FOR THE SP

- The examinee will name three objects for you and ask you to recall them after a few minutes. Pretend that you are unable to do so.
- If asked, give the examinee a list of your current medications (a piece of paper with nitroglycerin patch, hydrochlorothiazide, and aspirin written on it).
- Pretend that you have some weakness in your left arm.
- Show an increase in DTRs of the left arm and leg.

### CHALLENGING QUESTIONS TO ASK

"Do you think I have Alzheimer's disease?"

### SAMPLE EXAMINEE RESPONSE

"I don't know; we still need to do more testing. Tell me what you know about Alzheimer's disease."

## Examinee Checklist

### ENTRANCE:

☐ Examinee knocked on the door before entering.
☐ Examinee introduced self by name.
☐ Examinee identified his/her role or position.

☐ Examinee correctly used patient's name.

☐ Examinee made eye contact with the SP.

## HISTORY:

☐ Examinee showed compassion for your illness.

| ☑ Question | Patient Response |
|---|---|
| ☐ Chief complaint | Difficulty remembering things. |
| ☐ Onset | I can't remember exactly, but my daughter told me that I started forgetting last year. |
| ☐ Progression | My daughter has told me that it is getting worse. |
| ☐ Things that are difficult to remember | Turning off the stove, my phone number, my keys, the way to my home, the names of my friends. |
| ☐ Daily activities (bathing, feeding, toileting, dressing, transferring into and out of chairs and bed) | I have some trouble with these, and I need help sometimes. |
| ☐ Shopping | Well, I stopped shopping, since I've lost my way home so many times. My daughter shops for me. |
| ☐ Cooking | I stopped cooking because I often left the stove on and accidentally started a fire once. |
| ☐ Housework | My house is a mess; I keep forgetting where I put my stuff. |
| ☐ Paying the bills | My daughter does this for me. |
| ☐ Gait problems | No. |
| ☐ Urinary incontinence | No. |
| ☐ Feeling (sad, depressed) | I feel upset because of all of this. |
| ☐ Headaches | No. |
| ☐ Lightheadedness or feeling faint | Only if I stand up too quickly. |
| ☐ Passing out | No. |
| ☐ Falls | Yes, sometimes. |
| ☐ Head trauma | I think so; I had a large bruise on the side of my head a while back. |
| ☐ Did you see a doctor for that fall? | No, it was just a bruise. |
| ☐ Any shaking or seizures | No. |
| ☐ Visual changes | No. |
| ☐ Weakness/numbness/paresthesias | Yes, I have weakness in my left arm from a stroke I had a long time ago. |
| ☐ Speech difficulties | No. |
| ☐ Heart problems | I had a heart attack a long time ago. |

| ✓ | Question | Patient Response |
|---|----------|------------------|
| ☐ | Chest pain, shortness of breath, abdominal pain, nausea/vomiting, diarrhea/constipation | No. |
| ☐ | Weight changes | I've lost weight. I don't know how much. |
| ☐ | Appetite changes | I don't have an appetite. |
| ☐ | High blood pressure | Yes, for a long time. |
| ☐ | Current medications | I don't know their names. (Give the list to the examinee if he asks for it.) |
| ☐ | Past medical history | I think that's enough, isn't it? |
| ☐ | Past surgical history | I had a bowel obstruction a long time ago, and they removed part of my intestine. |
| ☐ | Family history | My father and mother died healthy a long time ago. |
| ☐ | Occupation | I retired after the death of my husband. |
| ☐ | Alcohol use | No. |
| ☐ | Illicit drug use | No. |
| ☐ | Tobacco | No. |
| ☐ | Social history | I live with my daughter. |
| ☐ | Sexual activity | Not since the death of my husband one year ago. |
| ☐ | Support systems (family, friends) | I have many friends who care about me, besides my daughter. |
| ☐ | Drug allergies | No. |

## Physical Examination:

- ☐ Examinee washed his/her hands.
- ☐ Examinee asked permission to start the exam.
- ☐ Examinee used respectful draping.
- ☐ Examinee did not repeat painful maneuvers.

| ✓ | Exam Component | Maneuver |
|---|----------------|----------|
| ☐ | Eye exam | Inspected pupils, fundus |
| ☐ | Neck exam | Carotid auscultation |
| ☐ | Pulmonary exam | Auscultation |
| ☐ | CV exam | Auscultation, orthostatic vital signs |
| ☐ | Abdominal exam | Palpation |
| ☐ | Neurologic exam | Mini-mental status exam, cranial nerves, motor exam, DTRs, gait, Romberg sign, sensory exam |

**Closure:**

☐ Examinee discussed initial diagnostic impressions.

☐ Examinee discussed initial management plans:

   ☐ Follow-up tests.

   ☐ Need to obtain history directly from other family members.

   ☐ Need to evaluate home safety and supervision.

   ☐ Community resources that help the patient at home.

   ☐ Offered support throughout her illness.

☐ Examinee asked if the patient has any other questions or concerns.

**USMLE**
**STEP 2 CS**

# PATIENT NOTE

**History**

**Physical Examination**

**Differential Diagnosis**

1.
2.
3.
4.
5.

**Diagnostic Workup**

1.
2.
3.
4.
5.

# PATIENT NOTE

## History

**HPI:** *65 yo F c/o difficulty remembering that started 1 year ago after the death of her husband and is getting progressively worse. This problem has affected her daily activities (bathing, feeding, toileting, dressing, transferring into and out of chairs and bed, shopping, cooking, managing money, using the telephone, cleaning the house). She has transient orthostatic lightheadedness and frequent falls, including at least 1 head injury for which she did not seek medical attention. The patient feels upset because of her difficulty. She has weight loss and no appetite. She denies headache, visual changes, gait problems, or urinary incontinence.*
**ROS:** *Residual weakness in her left arm after a stroke.*
**Allergies:** *NKDA.*
**Medications:** *HCTZ, aspirin, transdermal nitroglycerin.*
**PMH:** *Hypertension, stroke, MI. The patient cannot remember exactly when she had them.*
**PSH:** *Partial bowel resection due to obstruction many years ago.*
**SH:** *No smoking, no EtOH, no illicit drugs. She is a widow, is retired, lives with her daughter, and has a good support system (family, friends).*
**FH:** *Noncontributory.*

## Physical Examination

**VS:** *WNL, no orthostatic changes.*
**HEENT:** *Normocephalic, atraumatic, PERRLA, no funduscopic abnormalities.*
**Neck:** *Supple, no carotid bruits.*
**Chest:** *Clear breath sounds bilaterally.*
**Heart:** *RRR; normal S1/S2; no murmurs, rubs, or gallops.*
**Abdomen:** *Soft, nondistended, nontender, no hepatosplenomegaly.*
**Neuro:** Mental status: *Alert and oriented × 3, spells backward but can't recall 3 objects.* Cranial nerves: *2–12 intact.* Motor: *Strength 5/5 in all muscle groups except 3/5 in left arm.* DTRs: *Asymmetric 3+ in left upper and lower extremities, 1+ in the right,* ⊖*Babinski bilaterally.* Cerebellar: ⊖*Romberg.* Gait: *Normal.* Sensation: *Intact to pinprick and soft touch.*

## Differential Diagnosis

1. Alzheimer's disease
2. Vascular ("multi-infarct") dementia
3. Depression
4. Hypothyroidism
5. Vitamin $B_{12}$ deficiency
6. Subdural hematoma

## Diagnostic Workup

1. CBC
2. Electrolytes, calcium, glucose, BUN/Cr
4. Serum $B_{12}$, TSH, RPR
5. CT—head or MRI—brain
6. EEG or SPECT
7. Brain biopsy

## CASE DISCUSSION

### Differential Diagnosis

Dementia is an acquired, progressive impairment in cognitive function that includes amnesia plus some degree of aphasia, apraxia, agnosia, and/or impaired executive function. It is critical to obtain additional history from nondemented family members in order to establish an accurate time course of cognitive decline. The dementia syndromes are primarily clinical diagnoses reached after any partially reversible causes have been excluded.

- **Alzheimer's disease:** This is the most common cause of dementia. It usually has an insidious onset, with steady progressive decline in cognitive function over years. The earliest findings are impairment in memory and visuospatial abilities. Alzheimer's disease is a clinical diagnosis.
- **Vascular ("multi-infarct") dementia:** This often coexists with Alzheimer's disease, and given the patient's history of atherosclerotic vascular disease (e.g., stroke, MI), it could certainly be contributing in this case. There is classically more of a stepwise deterioration in vascular dementia compared to the steady cognitive decline seen in Alzheimer's. Also, there may be an earlier loss of executive function and personality changes in vascular dementia.
- **Depression:** The time course of cognitive decline following the death of the patient's husband may indicate depression, which can present atypically in the elderly and may mimic or more commonly coexist with dementia. However, it is more likely that her cognitive decline has been progressive for several years but became more noticeable to her children after her husband died.
- **Hypothyroidism:** This can cause neuropsychiatric symptoms (often a late finding) and must be ruled out in patients with dementia. However, there are no classic signs or symptoms to suggest hypothyroidism in this case.
- **Vitamin $B_{12}$ deficiency:** A prior bowel resection (e.g., of the terminal ileum) may put the patient at risk for this. It can cause depression, irritability, paranoia, confusion, and dementia but is usually associated with other neurologic symptoms, such as paresthesias and leg weakness. On occasion, dementia may precede the characteristic megaloblastic anemia.
- **Subdural hematoma:** This should be ruled out given the patient's history of falls and head trauma. Even though her cognitive decline spans at least a year, it is possible that a comorbid chronic subdural hematoma could have exacerbated her mental status changes in recent weeks or months.

### Diagnostic Workup

- **CBC:** To look for macrocytic anemia in vitamin $B_{12}$ deficiency.
- **Electrolytes, calcium, glucose, BUN/Cr:** To screen for medical conditions that can present with cognitive dysfunction (i.e., hypernatremia, hypercalcemia, hyperglycemia, uremia).
- **Serum $B_{12}$, TSH, RPR:** To screen for partially reversible causes of dementia (the latter can be restricted to patients manifesting signs of neurosyphilis).
- **CT–head:** To look for a crescent-shaped hypertense extra-axial mass in subdural hematoma, intracerebral masses, strokes, or dilated ventricles (as in normal pressure hydrocephalus).
- **MRI–brain:** Most sensitive exam to look for focal CNS lesions or atrophy.
- **EEG or SPECT:** Used in rare cases to help differentiate delirium from depression or dementia.
- **Brain biopsy:** Mainly used to rule out unusual entities such as Creutzfeldt-Jakob disease.

### Opening Scenario

Raymond Stern, a 56-year-old male, comes to the clinic for diabetes follow-up.

### Vital Signs

**BP:** 139/85 mmHg
**Temp:** 98.0°F (36.7°C)
**RR:** 15/minute
**HR:** 75/minute, regular

### Examinee Tasks

1. Take a focused history.
2. Perform a focused physical exam (do not perform rectal, genitourinary, or female breast exam).
3. Explain your clinical impression and workup plan to the patient.
4. Write the patient note after leaving the room.

### Checklist/SP Sheet

#### PATIENT DESCRIPTION

Patient is a 56 yo M.

#### NOTES FOR THE SP

- Pretend that you have a loss of sharp and dull sensations, vibration sense, and position sense in both feet ("stocking" distribution).
- Pretend to have a normal knee jerk and absent ankle reflex.

#### CHALLENGING QUESTIONS TO ASK

"Will I lose my feet, doctor?"

#### SAMPLE EXAMINEE RESPONSE

"Not if we continue to keep your blood sugars and cholesterol well controlled. The nerve damage to your feet is uncomfortable but alone will not lead to amputation as long as you take the proper measures to protect your feet from injury. We'll discuss how to do that later in the visit."

### Examinee Checklist

#### ENTRANCE:

☐ Examinee knocked on the door before entering.
☐ Examinee introduced self by name.
☐ Examinee identified his/her role or position.

☐   Examinee used patient's name.

☐   Examinee made eye contact with the SP.


**History:**

☐   Examinee showed compassion for your illness.


| ☑ *Question* | *Patient Response* |
| --- | --- |
| ☐ Chief complaint | I am here for a diabetes checkup. The last time I saw my doctor was six months ago. |
| ☐ Onset | I have had diabetes mellitus for the last 25 years. |
| ☐ Treatment | NPH insulin, 20 units in the morning and 15 units in the evening. |
| ☐ Compliance with medications | I never miss any doses. |
| ☐ Last blood sugar reading | Three days ago, and it was 135. |
| ☐ Blood sugar monitoring | I have a blood sugar monitor at home, and I check my blood sugar twice a week. It usually ranges between 120 and 145. |
| ☐ Last HgA$_{1c}$ | The last was six months ago, and it was 7. |
| ☐ Last time eyes were checked | One year ago, and there were no signs of diabetic eye disease. |
| ☐ How he is feeling today | Good. |
| ☐ Medication side effects | No. |
| ☐ Heart symptoms (chest pain, palpitations) | Sometimes I feel my heart racing, and I start sweating. |
| ☐ Description of these symptoms | It happens rarely if I miss a meal. I feel better after drinking orange juice. |
| ☐ Pulmonary complaints (shortness of breath, cough) | No. |
| ☐ Neurologic complaints (headaches, dizziness, weakness, numbness) | I have tingling and numbness in my feet all the time, especially at night; it's gotten worse over the past two months. |
| ☐ Polyuria, dysuria, hematuria | No. |
| ☐ Abdominal complaints (pain, dyspepsia, nausea) | No. |
| ☐ Change in bowel habits | No. |
| ☐ Visual problems (blurred vision) | No. |
| ☐ Foot infection | No. |
| ☐ Marital or work problems | No, my wife is great, and I am very happy in my job. |
| ☐ Feelings of anxiety or stress | No. |
| ☐ Weight changes | No. |
| ☐ Appetite changes | No. |

| ☑ Question | Patient Response |
|---|---|
| ☐ Hypertension | No. |
| ☐ History of hypercholesterolemia | Yes, it was diagnosed two years ago. |
| ☐ Previous heart problems | I had a heart attack last year. |
| ☐ History of TIA or stroke | No. |
| ☐ Current medications | Insulin, lovastatin, aspirin, atenolol. |
| ☐ Past medical history | Heart attack last year; high cholesterol for two years. |
| ☐ Past surgical history | None. |
| ☐ Family history | My father died at age 60 of a stroke. My mother is healthy. |
| ☐ Occupation | Clerk. |
| ☐ Diet | I eat everything that my wife cooks—meat, vegetables, etc. I don't follow any special diet. |
| ☐ Exercise | No. |
| ☐ Alcohol use | Yes, whiskey on the weekends. |
| ☐ CAGE questions | No (to all four). |
| ☐ Illicit drug use | No. |
| ☐ Tobacco | No. |
| ☐ Social history | I am married and live with my wife. |
| ☐ Sexual activity | I am not doing my job the way I used to, but my wife understands and is supportive. They told me it is the diabetes. Is it? |
| ☐ Type of sexual problem | I can't get it up, doc. I don't even wake up with erections anymore. |
| ☐ Libido | Good. |
| ☐ Duration | One or two years ago. |
| ☐ Feelings of depression | No. |
| ☐ Drug allergies | No. |

## Physical Examination:

☐ Examinee washed his/her hands.
☐ Examinee asked permission to start the exam.
☐ Examinee used respectful draping.
☐ Examinee did not repeat painful maneuvers.

| ☑ *Exam Component* | *Maneuver* |
|---|---|
| ☐ Eye exam | Funduscopic exam |
| ☐ Neck exam | Carotid auscultation |
| ☐ CV exam | Palpation, auscultation |
| ☐ Pulmonary exam | Auscultation |
| ☐ Abdominal exam | Auscultation, palpation, percussion |
| ☐ Extremities | Inspected feet, peripheral pulses |
| ☐ Neurologic exam | DTRs, Babinski's sign, sensation and strength in lower extremities |

## Closure:

☐ Examinee discussed initial diagnostic impressions.

☐ Examinee discussed initial management plans:

    ☐ Follow-up tests.

    ☐ Lifestyle modification (diet, exercise).

☐ Examinee asked if the patient has any other questions or concerns.

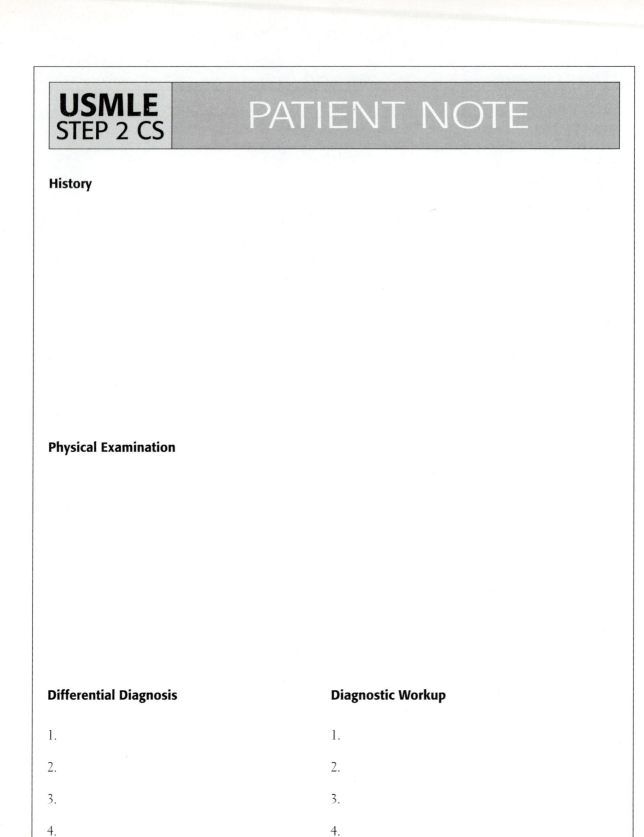

# USMLE STEP 2 CS

# PATIENT NOTE

**History**

**Physical Examination**

**Differential Diagnosis**

1.

2.

3.

4.

5.

**Diagnostic Workup**

1.

2.

3.

4.

5.

# PATIENT NOTE

## History

**HPI:** 56 yo M presents for diabetes follow-up. He has had diabetes mellitus for the last 25 years, treated with insulin. He is compliant with his medications and monitors his blood glucose level twice a week, with readings ranging between 120 and 145. His last HgA$_{1c}$ 6 months ago was 7%. He occasionally has episodes of palpitations and diaphoresis that occur after missing meals and resolve after drinking orange juice. He also has tingling and numbness in his feet all the time, especially at night, worsening over the last 2 months. No weight or appetite changes. Does not follow any special diet. Also notes loss of erections for 2 years.
**ROS:** Negative except as above.
**Allergies:** NKDA.
**Medications:** Lovastatin, NPH insulin, aspirin, atenolol.
**PMH:** Hypercholesterolemia diagnosed 2 years ago; MI 1 year ago.
**PSH:** None.
**SH:** No smoking, drinks whiskey on the weekends (CAGE 0/4), no illicit drugs. Works as a clerk. He is married and lives with his wife.
**FH:** Father died at age 60 of a stroke.

## Physical Examination

**VS:** WNL.
**HEENT:** PERRLA, no funduscopic abnormalities.
**Neck:** No carotid bruits, no JVD.
**Heart:** Apical impulse not displaced; RRR; normal S1/S2; no murmurs, rubs, or gallops.
**Chest:** Clear breath sounds bilaterally.
**Abdomen:** Soft, nondistended, nontender, ⊕BS, no bruits, no organomegaly.
**Extremities:** No edema, no skin breakdown, 2+ dorsalis pedis pulses.
**Neuro:** Motor: Strength 5/5 in bilateral lower extremities. DTRs: Symmetric 2+ knee jerks, absent ankle jerks and ⊖Babinski bilaterally. Sensation: Decreased pinprick; soft touch, vibratory, and position sense in bilateral lower extremities.

## Differential Diagnosis

1. Insulin-induced hypoglycemia
2. Peripheral neuropathy
   a. Diabetic peripheral neuropathy
   b. Alcoholic peripheral neuropathy
3. Multiple myeloma
4. Diabetic autonomic neuropathy, vascular disease, or medication-induced erectile dysfunction

## Diagnostic Workup

1. Genital exam
2. Serum glucose, HgA$_{1c}$
3. UA, urine microalbumin, BUN/Cr
4. CBC, SPEP
5. Doppler U/S—penis
6. Nerve conduction studies

## Case Discussion

### Differential Diagnosis

- **Insulin-induced hypoglycemia:** The patient's history suggests episodes of hypoglycemia. Typical signs and symptoms of hypoglycemia include sweating, tachycardia, palpitations, tremor, anxiety, weakness, confusion, and seizures. Maintaining tight glycemic control may occasionally result in hypoglycemia, and patients should be educated about how to recognize and treat this complication.
- **Peripheral neuropathy:** The differential for peripheral neuropathy includes hereditary, toxic, metabolic, infectious, inflammatory, and paraneoplastic disorders. No specific cause is determined in up 50% of cases. The history and exam guide us to some of the common causes discussed below.
  - **Diabetic peripheral neuropathy:** Involvement of the peripheral nervous system in diabetes may lead to symmetric sensory or mixed polyneuropathy (among other patterns of neuropathy). Burning foot paresthesias that are worse at night and loss of ankle reflexes, as seen in this case, are classic.
  - **Alcoholic peripheral neuropathy:** This causes a distal sensorimotor polyneuropathy marked by painful leg paresthesias and is directly attributable to alcohol or to associated nutritional deficiencies (e.g., thiamine and vitamin $B_{12}$).
- **Multiple myeloma:** Myeloma or other paraproteinemias must be ruled out in a patient with peripheral neuropathy.
- **Erectile dysfunction:** In diabetics, this is usually related to **vascular disease, autonomic neuropathy,** or **medications** (e.g., antihypertensives) for associated conditions. In general, impotence unaccompanied by loss of libido suggests either a vascular or a neurologic cause. Alcohol also causes an autonomic neuropathy and may contribute to erectile dysfunction.

### Diagnostic Workup

- **Genital exam:** To rule out Peyronie's disease (e.g., see penile scarring or plaque formation).
- **Serum glucose, HgA₁c:** To assess glycemic control.
- **UA, urine microalbumin, BUN/Cr:** To screen for diabetic nephropathy.
- **CBC, SPEP:** To detect paraproteinemias (e.g., multiple myeloma); anemia is often associated.
- **Doppler U/S–penis:** A helpful noninvasive test to measure penile blood flow.
- **Nerve conduction studies:** To confirm that symptoms arise from a peripheral nerve origin and to indicate an axonal vs. demyelinating mechanism.
- **Other studies:** In select cases, other studies useful in evaluating peripheral neuropathy include ESR, BUN/Cr, TSH, liver enzymes, RF, ANA, hepatitis B and C serologies, RPR, HIV antibody, urine heavy metal screen, CSF exam, CXR, and cutaneous nerve biopsy (e.g., to diagnose amyloidosis).

# CASE 14

## DOORWAY INFORMATION

### Opening Scenario

Edward Albright, a 53-year-old male, comes to the ER complaining of dizziness.

### Vital Signs

**BP:** 135/90 mmHg
**Temp:** 98.0°F (36.7°C)
**RR:** 16/minute
**HR:** 76/minute, regular

### Examinee Tasks

1. Take a focused history.
2. Perform a focused physical exam (do not perform rectal, genitourinary, or female breast exam).
3. Explain your clinical impression and workup plan to the patient.
4. Write the patient note after leaving the room.

### Checklist/SP Sheet

PATIENT DESCRIPTION

53 yo M, married with three children.

NOTES FOR THE SP

- Ask the examinee to speak loudly. Pretend that you have difficulty hearing in your left ear and that you hear him better when he talks close to your right ear.
- Refuse to walk if the examinee asks you to. Pretend that you are afraid of falling down. Walk only if the examinee explains why he would like to see your gait.

CHALLENGING QUESTIONS TO ASK

None.

### Examinee Checklist

ENTRANCE:

☐ Examinee knocked on the door before entering.
☐ Examinee introduced self by name.
☐ Examinee identified his/her role or position.
☐ Examinee correctly used patient's name.
☐ Examinee made eye contact with the SP.

HISTORY:

☐ Examinee showed compassion for your illness.

| ✓ | **Question** | **Patient Response** |
|---|---|---|
| ☐ | Chief complaint | I feel dizzy. |
| ☐ | Describe the meaning of dizziness | Well, I feel as if the room were spinning around me. |
| ☐ | Onset | Two days ago. |
| ☐ | Progression | It is getting worse. |
| ☐ | Constant/intermittent | It comes and goes. |
| ☐ | Duration | It lasts for 20–30 minutes. |
| ☐ | Timing | It can happen anytime. |
| ☐ | Positions that can elicit the dizziness (lying down, sitting, standing up) | When I get up from bed or lie down to sleep, but as I said, it can happen anytime. |
| ☐ | Positions that can relieve the dizziness | None. |
| ☐ | Tinnitus | No. |
| ☐ | Hearing loss (which ear, when) | Yes, I have difficulty hearing you in my left ear. This started yesterday. |
| ☐ | Fullness or pressure in the ears | No. |
| ☐ | Discharge from the ears | No. |
| ☐ | Falls | No, sometimes I feel unsteady as if I were going to fall down, but I don't fall. |
| ☐ | Nausea/vomiting | Yes, I feel nauseated and I vomited several times. |
| ☐ | Recent infections | I have had really bad diarrhea. I've had it for the past three days, but it is much better today. |
| ☐ | Fever | No. |
| ☐ | Stool | It was a watery diarrhea with no blood. |
| ☐ | Abdominal pain | No. |
| ☐ | URI (runny nose, sore throat, cough) | No. |
| ☐ | Headaches | No. |
| ☐ | Head trauma | No. |
| ☐ | Current medications | Furosemide, captopril. |
| ☐ | Past medical history | High blood pressure, diagnosed seven years ago. |
| ☐ | Past surgical history | Appendectomy. |
| ☐ | Family history | No similar problem in the family. |
| ☐ | Occupation | Executive director of an insurance company. |
| ☐ | Alcohol use | Yes, I drink 2–3 beers a week. |
| ☐ | Illicit drug use | No. |
| ☐ | Tobacco | No. |
| ☐ | Sexual activity | Yes, with my wife. |
| ☐ | Drug allergies | No. |

## Physical Examination:

☐ Examinee washed his/her hands.

☐ Examinee asked permission to start the exam.

☐ Examinee used respectful draping.

☐ Examinee did not repeat painful maneuvers.

| ☑ Exam Component | Maneuver |
|---|---|
| ☐ HEENT | Inspected for nystagmus, funduscopic exam, otoscopy, assessed hearing, Rinne and Weber tests, inspected mouth and throat |
| ☐ CV exam | Auscultation, orthostatic vital signs |
| ☐ Neurologic exam | Cranial nerves, motor exam, DTRs, gait, Romberg sign, tilt test (e.g., Dix-Hallpike maneuver) |

## Closure:

☐ Examinee discussed initial diagnostic impressions.

☐ Examinee discussed initial management plans:

    ☐ Follow-up tests.

☐ Examinee asked if the patient has any other questions or concerns.

# USMLE STEP 2 CS

# PATIENT NOTE

**History**

**Physical Examination**

**Differential Diagnosis**

1.

2.

3.

4.

5.

**Diagnostic Workup**

1.

2.

3.

4.

5.

## History

**HPI:** 53 yo M c/o intermittent dizziness that started 2 days ago. He feels the room spinning around him. The episodes occur at any time during the day, especially when he gets up from bed or lies down to sleep. They last for 20–30 minutes and are getting progressively worse. He has hearing loss in his left ear that started yesterday. He denies tinnitus, fullness in the ear, discharge, headache, or head trauma. No recent URI. He recalls having watery, nonbloody diarrhea over the past 3 days that resolved today.
**ROS:** Nausea and vomiting.
**Allergies:** NKDA.
**Medications:** Furosemide, captopril.
**PMH:** Hypertension, diagnosed 7 years ago.
**PSH:** Appendectomy.
**SH:** No smoking, 2–3 beers/week, no illicit drugs.
**FH:** Noncontributory.

## Physical Examination

**VS:** WNL, no orthostatic changes.
**HEENT:** NC/AT, PERRLA, EOMI without nystagmus, no papilledema, no cerumen, TMs normal, mouth and oropharynx normal.
**Heart:** RRR; normal S1/S2; no murmurs, rubs, or gallops.
**Neuro:** Cranial nerves: 2–12 grossly intact except for decreased hearing acuity in the left ear. Rinne positive (air conduction > bone conduction on the left), Weber no lateralization, ⊖tilt test. Motor: Strength 5/5 throughout. DTRs: 2+ intact, symmetric, ⊖Babinski bilaterally. Cerebellar: ⊖Romberg, finger to nose normal. Gait: Normal.

## Differential Diagnosis

1. Ménière's disease
2. Orthostatic hypotension due to dehydration
3. Benign paroxysmal positional vertigo
4. Labyrinthitis
5. Perilymphatic fistula
6. Acoustic neuroma

## Diagnostic Workup

1. Dix-Hallpike maneuver
2. RPR/VDRL
3. Audiometry
4. MRI—brain
5. Brain stem auditory evoked potentials
6. Electronystagmography

## CASE DISCUSSION

### Differential Diagnosis

Vertigo signals vestibular disease, whereas lightheadedness and dysequilibrium are usually nonvestibular in origin. A central vestibular system lesion (e.g., vertebrobasilar insufficiency, brain stem and cerebellar tumors, MS) is unlikely in this patient given the presence of hearing loss and an otherwise normal neurologic exam. Vertigo syndromes due to peripheral lesions are discussed below. These cases are often accompanied by nausea and vomiting, and vertigo may be so severe that the patient is unable to walk or stand.

- **Ménière's disease:** This classically presents with episodic vertigo (usually lasting 1–8 hours) and low-frequency hearing loss as well as with features not seen in this case, such as tinnitus and a sensation of aural fullness. Symptoms result from distention of the endolymphatic compartment of the inner ear. Syphilis and head trauma are two known causes.
- **Orthostatic hypotension due to dehydration:** Risk factors for dehydration in this case include diarrhea and loop diuretic use. However, the patient does not complain of lightheadedness and is not objectively orthostatic.
- **Benign paroxysmal positional vertigo (BPPV):** This describes transient vertigo following changes in head position but is not associated with hearing loss.
- **Labyrinthitis:** This frequently follows a viral infection (usually URI) and is accompanied by hearing loss and tinnitus, but vertigo is usually continuous and lasts several days to a week.
- **Perilymphatic fistula:** This is a rare cause of vertigo and sensorineural hearing loss, usually resulting from head trauma or extensive barotrauma. Episodes of vertigo are fleeting, generally lasting seconds.
- **Acoustic neuroma:** Acoustic neuroma more commonly causes continuous dysequilibrium rather than episodic vertigo. As noted above, central lesions are unlikely in patients with vertigo, hearing loss, and an otherwise normal neurologic exam. However, an intracranial mass lesion must be ruled out in any patient with unilateral hearing loss.

### Diagnostic Workup

- **Dix-Hallpike maneuver:** Used to diagnose BPPV (look for nystagmus, reproduction of vertigo).
- **RPR/VDRL:** To rule out syphilis, which can cause Ménière's disease.
- **Audiometry:** Useful to assess hearing function.
- **MRI—brain:** Required for the evaluation of central vestibular lesions.
- **Brain stem auditory evoked potentials:** Useful to help diagnose central vestibular disease.
- **Electronystagmography:** Useful to document characteristics of nystagmus that may differentiate central from peripheral vestibular system lesions.

## Opening Scenario

Gary Mitchell, a 46-year-old male, comes to the office complaining of fatigue.

## Vital Signs

BP: 120/85 mmHg
Temp: 98.2°F (36.8°C)
RR: 12/minute
HR: 65/minute, regular

## Examinee Tasks

1. Take a focused history.
2. Perform a focused physical exam (do not perform rectal, genitourinary, or female breast exam).
3. Explain your clinical impression and workup plan to the patient.
4. Write the patient note after leaving the room.

## Checklist/SP Sheet

PATIENT DESCRIPTION

Patient is a 46 yo M.

NOTES FOR THE SP

- Look sad, and don't smile.
- Speak and move slowly.
- Start yawning as the examinee enters the room.

CHALLENGING QUESTIONS TO ASK

- "I think that life is full of misery. Why do we have to live?"
- "I am afraid that I might have AIDS."

SAMPLE EXAMINEE RESPONSE

This patient clearly has more to say. Silence is appropriate here, or some small encouragement for the patient to continue talking. Alternatively, say, "It sounds as if you're losing hope. Have you thought about hurting yourself or tried to do so?" Or "Tell me more about your concern about AIDS."

## Examinee Checklist

ENTRANCE:

- ☐ Examinee knocked on the door before entering.
- ☐ Examinee introduced self by name.
- ☐ Examinee identified his/her role or position.

☐   Examinee correctly used patient's name.

☐   Examinee made eye contact with the SP.

### HISTORY:

☐   Examinee showed compassion for your illness.

☐   Examinee explored the patient's concern for AIDS (e.g., "Tell me more about that").

| ☑ Question | Patient Response |
|---|---|
| ☐ Chief complaint | Feeling tired, no energy. |
| ☐ Onset | Three months ago. |
| ☐ Associated events | We had a car accident, and I failed to save my friend from the car before it blew up. |
| ☐ Injuries related to the accident | No. |
| ☐ Progression of the fatigue during the day | Same throughout the day. |
| ☐ Affecting job/performance | Yes, I can't concentrate on my work anymore. I don't have the energy to work. |
| ☐ Appetite changes | Loss of appetite. |
| ☐ Weight changes | I have gained six pounds over the past three months. |
| ☐ Feeling of depression | Yes, I feel sad and depressed all the time. |
| ☐ Suicidal thoughts/plans/attempts | I think of death sometimes but have had no plans or attempts. |
| ☐ Feelings of blame or guilt | No, it was an accident. I tried to help my friend but couldn't. |
| ☐ Sleeping problems (falling asleep, staying asleep, early waking) | Well, I don't have problems falling asleep, but I wake up sometimes because of nightmares. I always see the accident, my friend calling for help, and the car blowing up. I feel so scared and helpless. I wake up very early in the morning and feel sleepy all day. |
| ☐ Snoring | Yes. |
| ☐ Loss of concentration | Yes, I can't concentrate on my work. |
| ☐ Associated symptoms (fever, chills, chest pain, shortness of breath, abdominal pain, diarrhea/constipation) | No. |
| ☐ Cold intolerance | Yes. |
| ☐ Skin/hair changes | My hair is falling out more than usual. |
| ☐ Current medications | None. |
| ☐ Past medical history | Well, I had some burning during urination. I don't really remember the diagnosis that the doctor reached, but it started with the letter C. I took antibiotics for one week. This was five months ago. |

| ✓ Question | Patient Response |
|---|---|
| ☐ Past surgical history | None. |
| ☐ Family history | My parents are alive and in good health. |
| ☐ Occupation | Accountant. |
| ☐ Alcohol use | Two to three beers a month. |
| ☐ Illicit drug use | Never. |
| ☐ Tobacco | One pack a day for 25 years. |
| ☐ Exercise | No. |
| ☐ Diet | The usual. I haven't changed anything in my diet in more than 10 years. |
| ☐ Sexual activity | Not interested anymore. I have a girlfriend, and we have been together for the last six months. I don't use condoms because they make me feel uncomfortable. I have had several sexual partners in the past. |
| ☐ Drug allergies | No. |

## Physical Examination:

☐ Examinee washed his/her hands.
☐ Examinee asked permission to start the exam.
☐ Examinee used respectful draping.
☐ Examinee did not repeat painful maneuvers.

| ✓ Exam Component | Maneuver |
|---|---|
| ☐ Head and neck exam | Inspected conjunctivae, mouth and throat, lymph nodes; examined thyroid gland |
| ☐ CV exam | Auscultation |
| ☐ Pulmonary exam | Auscultation |
| ☐ Abdominal exam | Auscultation, palpation, and percussion |
| ☐ Extremities | Inspection, checked DTRs |

## Closure:

☐ Examinee discussed initial diagnostic impressions.
☐ Examinee discussed initial management plans:
    ☐ Diagnostic tests.
    ☐ Lifestyle modification (diet, exercise, relaxation techniques, smoking cessation).
    ☐ Discussed safe sex practices.

☐ Discussed HIV testing and consent.

☐ Depression counseling:

☐ Helped the patient identify sources of support (e.g., trusted friends and loved ones) and provided information about community groups.

☐ Discussed the possible need for referral to a psychiatrist.

☐ Suicide contract (contact your physician or go to the ER for any suicidal thoughts or plans).

☐ Examinee asked if the patient has any other questions or concerns.

**USMLE** STEP 2 CS

# PATIENT NOTE

**History**

**Physical Examination**

**Differential Diagnosis**

1.
2.
3.
4.
5.

**Diagnostic Workup**

1.
2.
3.
4.
5.

## History

**HPI:** 46 yo M c/o fatigue. The patient notes that this fatigue began 3 months ago, following an unsuccessful attempt to save his friend after a car accident. The fatigue is constant throughout the day. He has low energy and decreased ability to concentrate, which have adversely affected his job as an accountant. Over the past 3 months, the patient had a decrease in appetite but gained 6 pounds. He feels sleepy throughout the day, wakes up early in the morning, and has difficulty staying asleep because of recurrent nightmares about the accident. He also reports snoring. The patient can't tolerate cold weather and complains of hair loss. He denies constipation. He has lost his interest in sex and admits to being depressed and helpless, with suicidal thoughts but no plans or attempts. The patient denies feelings of blame or guilt.

**ROS:** Negative except as above.

**Allergies:** NKDA.

**Medications:** None.

**PMH:** Urethritis (possibly chlamydia), treated 5 months ago.

**SH:** One PPD for 25 years, 2 beers/month. History of unprotected sex with multiple female partners.

**FH:** Noncontributory.

## Physical Examination

Patient is in no acute distress, looks tired with a flat affect, speaks and moves slowly.

**VS:** WNL.

**HEENT:** No conjunctival pallor, mouth and pharynx WNL.

**Neck:** No lymphadenopathy, thyroid normal.

**Chest:** Clear breath sounds bilaterally.

**Heart:** RRR; normal S1/S2; no murmurs, rubs, or gallops.

**Abdomen:** Soft, nondistended, nontender, ⊕BS, no hepatosplenomegaly.

**Extremities:** No edema, normal DTRs in lower extremities.

## Differential Diagnosis

1. Depression
2. Adjustment disorder with depressed mood
3. Hypothyroidism
4. Obstructive sleep apnea
5. Post-traumatic stress disorder
6. HIV infection

## Diagnostic Workup

1. CBC
2. TSH
3. Ambulatory nocturnal pulse oximetry
4. Polysomnography
5. HIV antibody
6. MRI—brain

## CASE DISCUSSION

### Differential Diagnosis

Fatigue is a common, nonspecific complaint with many etiologies, from simple overexertion to serious diseases such as cancer.

- **Depression:** Many classic symptoms are present in this patient. The mnemonic **SIG EM CAPS** helps recall them: Sleep disturbance, decreased Interest, feelings of Guilt, decreased Energy, depressed Mood, decreased Concentration, change in Appetite, Psychomotor agitation or slowing, and Suicidal ideation.
- **Adjustment disorder with depressed mood:** The stress of witnessing a friend's death may lead to maladaptive behavior, with depression as the predominant symptom.
- **Hypothyroidism:** This should be ruled out in a patient with fatigue for months. The cold intolerance, hair loss, and weight gain are additional nonspecific symptoms that suggest this diagnosis.
- **Obstructive sleep apnea:** Although the patient snores, this diagnosis is less likely given that his excessive daytime somnolence is occurring in the context of many other depressive symptoms. Nonetheless, obstructive sleep apnea is common and underdiagnosed, and it does occur in nonobese patients.
- **Post-traumatic stress disorder (PTSD):** This is characterized by (1) reexperiencing a traumatic event (e.g., flashbacks); (2) avoidance of stimuli associated with the trauma; and (3) increased arousal (e.g., anxiety, sleep disturbance, hypervigilance). Despite having nightmares about the accident, this patient does not sufficiently manifest the last two features of the disorder.
- **HIV infection:** Given his history of STDs, the patient should also be tested for this. However, it is highly unlikely that HIV infection accounts for his current depression (unless there are frontal lobe lesions due to infection or malignancy).

### Diagnostic Workup

- **CBC:** To rule out anemia.
- **TSH:** A screening test for hypothyroidism.
- **Ambulatory nocturnal pulse oximetry:** An initial test to evaluate possible obstructive sleep apnea.
- **Polysomnography:** To diagnose obstructive sleep apnea.
- **HIV antibody:** To rule out HIV infection.
- **MRI–brain:** To rule out the exceedingly rare possibility that the patient's symptoms are due to an intracranial mass lesion.

# CASE 16

## DOORWAY INFORMATION

### Opening Scenario

Jessica Lee, a 32-year-old female, comes to the office complaining of fatigue.

### Vital Signs

**BP:** 120/85 mmHg
**Temp:** 98.2°F (36.8°C)
**RR:** 13/minute
**HR:** 80/minute, regular

### Examinee Tasks

1. Take a focused history.
2. Perform a focused physical exam (do not perform rectal, genitourinary, or female breast exam).
3. Explain your clinical impression and workup plan to the patient.
4. Write the patient note after leaving the room.

### Checklist/SP Sheet

PATIENT DESCRIPTION

Patient is a 32 yo F, married with two children.

NOTES FOR THE SP

- Look anxious and pale.
- Exhibit bruises on the face and arms that elicit pain when touched.

CHALLENGING QUESTIONS TO ASK

"I am drinking a lot of water, doctor. What do you think the reason is?"

SAMPLE EXAMINEE RESPONSE

"I don't know for sure, but I want to run some tests. We need to make sure that you haven't developed diabetes."

### Examinee Checklist

ENTRANCE:

- ☐ Examinee knocked on the door before entering.
- ☐ Examinee introduced self by name.
- ☐ Examinee identified his/her role or position.
- ☐ Examinee correctly used patient's name.
- ☐ Examinee made eye contact with the SP.

HISTORY:

- ☐ Examinee showed compassion for your illness.

| ☑ Question | Patient Response |
|---|---|
| ☐ Chief complaint | Feeling tired, weak, no energy. |
| ☐ Onset | Five months ago. |
| ☐ Associated events | None. |
| ☐ Progression of the fatigue during the day | I feel okay in the morning; then gradually I start feeling more and more tired and weak. |
| ☐ Change in vision (double vision) during the day | No. |
| ☐ Affecting job/performance | Yes, I don't have energy to work. |
| ☐ Appetite changes | I have a very good appetite. |
| ☐ Weight changes | No. |
| ☐ Feeling of depression | Sometimes I feel sad. |
| ☐ Cause of bruises | I fell down the stairs and hurt myself (looks anxious). It is my fault. I don't always pay attention. |
| ☐ Being physically or emotionally hurt or abused by anybody | Well, sometimes when my husband gets angry with me, but he loves me very much, and he promises not to do it again. |
| ☐ Feeling safe/afraid at home | Sometimes I feel afraid, especially when my husband gets drunk. |
| ☐ Are the children being abused or threatened? | Well, he slapped my younger son the other day for breaking a glass. He should be more attentive. |
| ☐ Suicidal thoughts/plans/attempts | No. |
| ☐ Feelings of blame or guilt | Yes, I think I am being awkward. It is my fault. |
| ☐ Presence of guns at home | No. |
| ☐ Any family members who know about the abuse | No. |
| ☐ Emergency plan | No. |
| ☐ Sleeping problems (falling asleep, staying asleep, early waking, snoring) | No. |
| ☐ Loss of concentration | Yes, I can't concentrate on my work. |
| ☐ Menstrual period | Regular and heavy; lasts seven days. |
| ☐ Last menstrual period | Two weeks ago. |
| ☐ Urinary symptoms | I recently started to wake up at night to urinate. |
| ☐ Polyuria | Yes, I have to go to the bathroom more often during the day. |
| ☐ Pain during urination or change in the color of urine | No. |
| ☐ Polydipsia | Yes, I feel thirsty all the time, and I drink a lot of water. |
| ☐ Associated symptoms (fever, chills, chest pain, shortness of breath, abdominal pain, diarrhea/constipation, cold intolerance, skin/hair changes) | None. |

| ✓ Question | Patient Response |
|---|---|
| ☐ Current medications | None. |
| ☐ Past medical history | None. |
| ☐ Past surgical history | I fell and broke my arm a year ago. |
| ☐ Family history | My father had diabetes and died of a heart attack. My mother is in a nursing home with Alzheimer's. |
| ☐ Occupation | Nurse. |
| ☐ Alcohol use | No. |
| ☐ Illicit drug use | Never. |
| ☐ Tobacco | No. |
| ☐ Exercise | No. |
| ☐ Diet | I am a vegetarian. |
| ☐ Sexual activity | I don't feel any desire for sex, but we do it when my husband wants. |
| ☐ Drug allergies | No. |

## Physical Examination:

☐ Examinee washed his/her hands.
☐ Examinee asked permission to start the exam.
☐ Examinee used respectful draping.
☐ Examinee did not repeat painful maneuvers.

| ✓ Exam Component | Maneuver |
|---|---|
| ☐ Head and neck exam | Inspected conjunctivae, mouth and throat, lymph nodes; examined thyroid gland |
| ☐ CV exam | Auscultation |
| ☐ Pulmonary exam | Auscultation |
| ☐ Abdominal exam | Auscultation, palpation, and percussion |
| ☐ Extremities | Inspection, motor exam, DTRs |

## Closure:

☐ Examinee discussed initial diagnostic impressions.
☐ Examinee discussed initial management plans:
    ☐ Diagnostic tests.
    ☐ Domestic violence counseling:
        ☐ "I care about your safety and I am always available for help and support."
        ☐ "Everything we discuss is confidential, but I must involve child protective services if your children are being abused."
        ☐ Support group information, including contact numbers or Web sites.
        ☐ Safety planning.
☐ Examinee asked if the patient has any other questions or concerns.

**USMLE**
STEP 2 CS

# PATIENT NOTE

**History**

**Physical Examination**

**Differential Diagnosis**

1.
2.
3.
4.
5.

**Diagnostic Workup**

1.
2.
3.
4.
5.

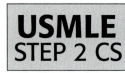

# PATIENT NOTE

## History

**HPI:** 32 yo F c/o fatigue and weakness. The patient notes that the fatigue and weakness started 5 months ago. The fatigue increases gradually during the day. She complains of loss of energy and concentration that adversely affects her job as a nurse. After questioning about the bruises on her face and arms, she admits that her husband, who is an alcoholic, has beaten her. She also reports at least 1 episode of physical abuse directed at her youngest son. She tries to defend his actions, feels guilty, and blames herself. She has not reported this to anyone and has no emergency plan. She feels sad but denies suicidal ideation. The patient also complains of polyuria, polydipsia, and nocturia that also began 5 months ago. She denies burning on urination or change in the color of urine. Her last menstrual period was 2 weeks ago; the menstrual period is regular, q28 days, lasting for 7 days of heavy flow. No constipation, cold intolerance, or change in appetite or weight. No sleep problems.
**ROS:** Negative except as above.
**Allergies:** NKDA.
**Medications:** None.
**SH:** No smoking, no EtOH. Sexually active with her husband; decreased sexual desire.
**FH:** Diabetic father died from a heart attack; mother is in a nursing home with Alzheimer's disease.

## Physical Examination

Patient is in no acute distress, looks anxious.
**VS:** WNL.
**HEENT:** Pale conjunctivae.
**Neck:** No lymphadenopathy, thyroid normal.
**Chest:** Clear breath sounds bilaterally.
**Heart:** RRR; normal S1/S2; no murmurs, rubs, or gallops.
**Abdomen:** Soft, nondistended, nontender, ⊕BS, no hepatosplenomegaly.
**Extremities:** Muscle strength 5/5 throughout; DTRs 2+; symmetric, painful bruises on both arms.

## Differential Diagnosis

1. Domestic violence
2. Depression
3. Diabetes mellitus
4. Diabetes insipidus
5. Anemia
6. Myasthenia gravis
7. Hypothyroidism

## Diagnostic Workup

1. CBC, iron level, TIBC, ferritin, serum $B_{12}$
2. Electrolytes
3. UA
4. Serum glucose, $HgA_{1c}$
5. TSH
6. MRI—brain (pituitary protocol)
7. DDAVP nasal spray test (vasopressin)

## CASE DISCUSSION

### Differential Diagnosis

- **Domestic violence:** The patient is clearly a victim of domestic violence and of her husband's alcoholism. This can explain many of her symptoms but not the polyuria and polydipsia.
- **Depression:** As above, depression likely coexists but does not account for the patient's recent polyuria and polydipsia (if objectively verified).
- **Diabetes mellitus (DM):** Aside from domestic violence issues, many of the patient's symptoms can be explained by new-onset diabetes. Her positive family history puts her at risk. She should also be asked about any recent vaginal yeast infections, which are a frequent complication of hyperglycemia (and may be its initial presenting symptom).
- **Diabetes insipidus (DI):** This is an uncommon disease characterized by polyuria (of low specific gravity) and polydipsia. It has many etiologies and is caused by a deficiency of or resistance to vasopressin.
- **Anemia:** This may also help explain her fatigue and weakness. Menstruating females often have an iron-deficiency anemia, and strict vegans may also have anemia related to vitamin $B_{12}$ deficiency. Conjunctival pallor on exam has a high likelihood ratio for predicting a hematocrit < 30% (hemoglobin < 10 g/dL).
- **Myasthenia gravis:** Increasing fatigue as the day progresses is highly nonspecific. By contrast, this disease involves fluctuating muscle weakness and presents with ptosis, diplopia, difficulty in chewing or swallowing, respiratory difficulties, and/or limb weakness.
- **Hypothyroidism:** Nonspecific symptoms such as fatigue and weakness may suggest this common diagnosis. However, hypothyroidism does not explain polyuria, polydipsia, or the admitted physical abuse.

### Diagnostic Workup

- **CBC, iron level, TIBC, ferritin, serum $B_{12}$:** Blood tests to investigate anemia.
- **Electrolytes:** May see hypernatremia in DI.
- **UA:** Dilute urine is seen in DI, glycosuria in DM.
- **Serum glucose, HgA$_{1c}$:** To screen for DM.
- **TSH:** Must rule out thyroid disease in a patient with symptoms of depression.
- **MRI—brain (pituitary protocol):** To look for mass lesions in central DI.
- **DDAVP nasal spray test ("vasopressin challenge test"):** To confirm a clinical suspicion of central DI.

## Opening Scenario

William Jordan, a 61-year-old male, comes to the office complaining of fatigue.

## Vital Signs

BP: 135/85 mmHg
Temp: 98.6°F (37°C)
RR: 13/minute
HR: 70/minute, regular

## Examinee Tasks

1. Take a focused history.
2. Perform a focused physical exam (do not perform rectal, genitourinary, or female breast exam).
3. Explain your clinical impression and workup plan to the patient.
4. Write the patient note after leaving the room.

## Checklist/SP Sheet

### PATIENT DESCRIPTION

61 yo M, married with three children.

### NOTES FOR THE SP

- Look weak and sad, and sit leaning forward.
- Exhibit abdominal discomfort that increases when you lie on your back.
- Show pain on palpation of the epigastric area.

### CHALLENGING QUESTIONS TO ASK

"I want to go on a trip with my wife. Can we do the tests after I come back?"

### SAMPLE EXAMINEE RESPONSE

"It doesn't sound as if you're feeling well enough to be able to enjoy a trip. Let's do some initial blood tests, and then we can see how you're feeling and decide whether we're comfortable letting you go away."

## Examinee Checklist

### ENTRANCE:

☐ Examinee knocked on the door before entering.
☐ Examinee introduced self by name.
☐ Examinee identified his/her role or position.
☐ Examinee correctly used patient's name.
☐ Examinee made eye contact with the SP.

## HISTORY:

☐   Examinee showed compassion for your illness.

| ☑ Question | Patient Response |
|---|---|
| ☐ Chief complaint | Feeling tired, weak, low energy. |
| ☐ Onset | Six months ago. |
| ☐ Associated events | None. |
| ☐ Progression of the fatigue during the day | The same throughout the day. |
| ☐ Affecting job/performance | Yes, I don't have energy for my daily 30-minute walk with my dog, and even at work I am not as energetic as before. |
| ☐ Appetite changes | I have a poor appetite. |
| ☐ Weight changes | I lost eight pounds during the past six months. |
| ☐ Change in bowel habits | No, I have a bowel movement twice or three times a week. It has been like this for the last 10 years. |
| ☐ Blood in stool | No. |
| ☐ Abdominal pain or discomfort | Yes, I do feel some discomfort here (points to the epigastric area). |
| ☐ Onset of discomfort | Four months ago; it increased gradually. |
| ☐ Quality | Vague, deep. |
| ☐ Severity on a scale | 4/10. |
| ☐ Alleviating/exacerbating factors | Nothing makes it worse, but I feel better when I lean forward. |
| ☐ Relationship to food | No. |
| ☐ Radiation | I feel the discomfort reaching my back. |
| ☐ Nausea/vomiting | Sometimes I feel nauseated. |
| ☐ Feeling of depression | Yes, I feel sad. |
| ☐ Reason for feeling sad | I don't know, really. |
| ☐ Suicidal thoughts/plans/attempts | No. |
| ☐ Feelings of blame, guilt, worthlessness | No. |
| ☐ Sleeping problems (falling asleep, staying asleep, early waking, snoring) | I wake up unusually early in the morning. It has been like this for the past two months. |
| ☐ Loss of concentration | Yes, I can't concentrate anymore while watching the news or playing cards with my friends. |
| ☐ Loss of interest | I don't enjoy playing cards with my friends anymore. I feel that life is boring. |

| ☑ *Question* | *Patient Response* |
|---|---|
| ☐ Associated symptoms (fever/chills, chest pain, cough, shortness of breath, cold intolerance, skin/hair changes) | None. |
| ☐ Current medications | Tylenol, but it is not helping. |
| ☐ Past psychiatric history | No. |
| ☐ Past medical history | No. |
| ☐ Past surgical history | Appendectomy at age 16. |
| ☐ Family history | My father died in a car accident and had diabetes, and my mother died of breast cancer. |
| ☐ Occupation | Police officer, retired one year ago. |
| ☐ Alcohol use | One or two beers 2–3 times a week. |
| ☐ Illicit drug use | Never. |
| ☐ Tobacco | I stopped it six months ago after 30 years of smoking one pack a day (because I felt disgusted, and smoking made me feel sick). |
| ☐ Exercise | I walk 30 minutes every day. |
| ☐ Diet | Regular; I like junk food. |
| ☐ Sexual activity | Sexually active with my wife. |
| ☐ Drug allergies | No. |

## Physical Examination:

- ☐ Examinee washed his/her hands.
- ☐ Examinee asked permission to start the exam.
- ☐ Examinee used respectful draping.
- ☐ Examinee did not repeat painful maneuvers.

| ☑ *Exam Component* | *Maneuver* |
|---|---|
| ☐ Head and neck exam | Inspected conjunctivae, mouth and throat, lymph nodes; examined thyroid gland |
| ☐ CV exam | Auscultation |
| ☐ Pulmonary exam | Auscultation |
| ☐ Abdominal exam | Auscultation, percussion, palpation (including rebound tenderness and Murphy's sign). |
| ☐ Extremities | Inspection, palpation |

**Closure:**

☐ Examinee discussed initial diagnostic impressions.

☐ Examinee discussed initial management plans:

    ☐ Diagnostic tests.

    ☐ Depression counseling:

        ☐ Asked about patient's existing support system (friends, family).

        ☐ Discussed available support systems in the hospital and community.

        ☐ Coping skills: Exercise, relaxation techniques, spending more time with family and friends.

☐ Examinee asked if the patient has any other questions or concerns.

**USMLE**
STEP 2 CS

# PATIENT NOTE

**History**

**Physical Examination**

**Differential Diagnosis**

1.

2.

3.

4.

5.

**Diagnostic Workup**

1.

2.

3.

4.

5.

## History

**HPI:** 61 yo M c/o fatigue and weakness. The patient notes that the fatigue and weakness started 6 months ago. He feels tired all day. He has poor appetite and lost 8 pounds in the last 6 months. He also complains of occasional nausea and of a vague, deep epigastric discomfort that radiates to the back. This discomfort started 4 months ago and has gradually increased to a severity of 4/10. The discomfort decreases when he leans forward and increases when he lies on his back. There is no relationship of the pain to food. No change in bowel movements or blood in the stool. He feels sad sometimes, has lost interest in things that he used to enjoy, wakes up unusually early in the morning, and complains of low energy and concentration that have affected his daily activities and work. The patient denies suicidal ideation or plans. No feelings of guilt or worthlessness.

**ROS:** Negative except as above.

**Allergies:** NKDA.

**Medications:** Tylenol.

**PMH:** None.

**PSH:** Appendectomy at age 16.

**SH:** One PPD for 30 years; stopped 6 months ago. Drinks 1–2 beers 2–3 times/week. Sexually active with his wife.

**FH:** Father with diabetes, died accidentally. Mother died from breast cancer.

## Physical Examination

Patient is in no acute distress, looks sad.

**VS:** WNL.

**HEENT:** No conjunctival pallor, mouth and pharynx normal.

**Neck:** Supple, no JVD, no lymphadenopathy, thyroid normal.

**Chest:** Clear breath sounds bilaterally.

**Heart:** RRR; normal S1/S2; no murmurs, rubs, or gallops.

**Abdomen:** Soft, nondistended, mild epigastric tenderness, no rebound tenderness, ⊖Murphy's, ⊕BS, no hepatosplenomegaly.

**Extremities:** No edema.

## Differential Diagnosis

1. Depression
2. Pancreatic cancer
3. Chronic pancreatitis
4. Peptic ulcer disease
5. Hypothyroidism

## Diagnostic Workup

1. CBC, stool for occult blood
2. Glucose
3. Amylase, lipase
4. AST/ALT/bilirubin/alkaline phosphatase
5. TSH
6. AXR
7. CT or U/S—abdomen
8. Stool for fecal fat
9. Tumor markers (CEA, CA 19-9)
10. Upper endoscopy
11. Barium upper GI study

## CASE DISCUSSION

### Differential Diagnosis

- **Depression:** The patient has many classic symptoms of depression (**SIG EM CAPS**; see Case 15). Although it may be a somatic symptom of depression, his abdominal pain is of significant concern and warrants a thorough medical evaluation.
- **Pancreatic cancer:** The pattern and location of pain are worrisome for pancreatic disease, and weight loss raises a concern for malignancy. Depression may be its initial manifestation. Diarrhea, presumably due to malabsorption, is also an occasional early finding (not seen in this case).
- **Chronic pancreatitis:** The pattern and location of pain are consistent with this diagnosis, but usually there is a history of recurrent episodes of similar pain. The patient's alcohol use should be explored further, as alcoholism accounts for 70–80% of chronic pancreatitis.
- **Peptic ulcer disease:** Suspect this diagnosis in any patient with epigastric pain, although the complaint is neither sensitive nor specific enough to make a reliable diagnosis. It is important to note that many patients deny any relationship of the pain to meals. Weight loss, however, is unusual in uncomplicated ulcer disease and may suggest gastric malignancy.
- **Hypothyroidism:** Nonspecific symptoms such as fatigue and weakness may suggest this common diagnosis. Abdominal pain is unusual.

### Diagnostic Workup

- **CBC, stool for occult blood:** To screen for blood loss in peptic ulcer.
- **Glucose:** To screen for pancreatic endocrine dysfunction (i.e., diabetes mellitus).
- **Amylase, lipase:** Nonspecific, but can be elevated in chronic pancreatitis or malignancy.
- **AST/ALT/bilirubin/alkaline phosphatase:** To look for evidence of obstructive jaundice (often seen in pancreatic cancer).
- **TSH:** Thyroid disease must be ruled out in a patient with symptoms of depression.
- **AXR:** To look for pancreatic calcification in chronic pancreatitis.
- **CT or U/S—abdomen:** To diagnose pancreatic cancer or other pathology.
- **Stool for fecal fat:** To look for evidence of pancreatic exocrine insufficiency.
- **Tumor markers (e.g., CEA, CA 19-9):** Nonspecific; mainly useful in following therapy for established cancers.
- **Upper endoscopy:** To diagnose ulcer disease.
- **Barium upper GI study:** To diagnose peptic ulcer disease and esophagitis (used less frequently now).

## Opening Scenario

Kelly Clark, a 35-year-old female, comes to the ER complaining of headache.

## Vital Signs

**BP:** 135/90 mmHg
**Temp:** 98.6°F (37°C)
**RR:** 16/minute
**HR:** 76/minute, regular

## Examinee Tasks

1. Take a focused history.
2. Perform a focused physical exam (do not perform rectal, genitourinary, or female breast exam).
3. Explain your clinical impression and workup plan to the patient.
4. Write the patient note after leaving the room.

## Checklist/SP Sheet

PATIENT DESCRIPTION

Patient is a 35 yo F, married with three children.

NOTES FOR THE SP

Hold the right side of your head during the encounter and look as if you are in severe pain.

CHALLENGING QUESTIONS TO ASK

"Do you have anything that will make me feel better? Please, doctor, I am in pain."

SAMPLE EXAMINEE RESPONSE

"Yes, we have many options for medicines to relieve your pain, but first I need to learn as much as I can about your pain so that I can recommend the best medicine."

## Examinee Checklist

ENTRANCE:

☐ Examinee knocked on the door before entering.
☐ Examinee introduced self by name.
☐ Examinee identified his/her role or position.
☐ Examinee correctly used patient's name.
☐ Examinee made eye contact with the SP.

HISTORY:

☐ Examinee showed compassion for your pain.

| ☑ | Question | Patient Response |
|---|---|---|
| ☐ | Chief complaint | Headache. |
| ☐ | Onset | Two weeks ago. |
| ☐ | Constant/intermittent | Well, I don't have the pain all the time. It comes and goes. |
| ☐ | Frequency | At least once a day. |
| ☐ | Progression | It is getting worse (2–3 times a day). |
| ☐ | Severity on a scale | When I have the pain, it is 9/10 and prevents me from working. |
| ☐ | Location | It is here (points to the whole right side of the head). |
| ☐ | Duration | One or two hours. |
| ☐ | Radiation (changes its location) | No. |
| ☐ | Quality | Sharp and pounding. |
| ☐ | Aura (warning that the headache is about to come) | No. |
| ☐ | Timing (the same time every day/ morning/evening) | The headache may come at any time. I'm having one now. |
| ☐ | Relationship with menses | No. |
| ☐ | Alleviating factors | Resting in a quiet, dark room; sleep, aspirin. |
| ☐ | Exacerbating factors | Stress, light, and noise. |
| ☐ | Nausea/vomiting | Sometimes I feel nauseated when I am in pain. Yesterday I vomited for the first time. |
| ☐ | Headache wakes you up from sleep | No. |
| ☐ | Visual changes/tears/red eye | No. |
| ☐ | Weakness/numbness | No. |
| ☐ | Speech difficulties | No. |
| ☐ | Runny nose during the attack | No. |
| ☐ | Similar episodes before | Yes, in college I had a similar headache that was accompanied by nausea. |
| ☐ | Weight/appetite changes | No. |
| ☐ | Joint pain/fatigue | Occasional aches and pains treated with ibuprofen. |
| ☐ | Stress | Yes, I am working on a new project that I have to finish this month. Last month was a disaster. I worked hard on my designs, but they were rejected, and I have to start all over again. |
| ☐ | Head trauma | No. |
| ☐ | Last menstrual period | Two weeks ago. |
| ☐ | Current medications | Ibuprofen. |

| ☑ **Question** | **Patient Response** |
| --- | --- |
| ☐ Past medical history | An episode of sinusitis four months ago, treated with amoxicillin (but the pain was different from the one I have now). |
| ☐ Past surgical history | Tubal ligation eight years ago. |
| ☐ Family history | My father died at age 65 of a brain tumor. My mother is alive and has migraines. |
| ☐ Occupation | Engineer. |
| ☐ Alcohol use | No. |
| ☐ Illicit drug use | No. |
| ☐ Tobacco use | No. |
| ☐ Social history | I live with my husband and three children. |
| ☐ Sexual activity | With my husband. |
| ☐ Use of OCPs | No, I had a tubal ligation after my third child eight years ago. |
| ☐ Drug allergies | No. |

## Physical Examination:

☐ Examinee washed his/her hands.
☐ Examinee asked permission to start the exam.
☐ Examinee used respectful draping.
☐ Examinee did not repeat painful maneuvers.

| ☑ **Exam Component** | **Maneuver** |
| --- | --- |
| ☐ HEENT | Palpation (head, facial sinuses, temporomandibular joints), funduscopic exam; inspected nose, mouth, teeth, and throat |
| ☐ Neck | Inspection, palpation |
| ☐ CV exam | Auscultation |
| ☐ Pulmonary exam | Auscultation |
| ☐ Neurologic exam | Cranial nerves, muscle strength, DTRs |

## Closure:

☐ Examinee discussed initial diagnostic impressions.
☐ Examinee discussed initial management plans.
☐ Examinee asked if the patient has any other questions or concerns.

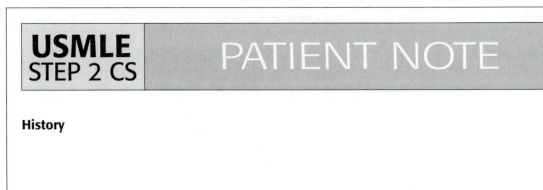

**History**

**Physical Examination**

**Differential Diagnosis**

1.

2.

3.

4.

5.

**Diagnostic Workup**

1.

2.

3.

4.

5.

PRACTICE CASES

## History

**HPI:** 35 yo F c/o daily headaches for 2 weeks. These headaches occur 2–3 times a day and last for 1–2 hours. The pain is sharp and pounding. It is located on the right hemisphere of the head, with no radiation or preceding aura. The pain reaches 9/10 in severity and prevents the patient from continuing her activities. Headaches are exacerbated by stress, light, and noise and are alleviated by resting in a dark room, sleep, and aspirin. The pain is sometimes accompanied by nausea and vomiting. No changes in weight and appetite.
**ROS:** Occasional aches and pains.
**Allergies:** NKDA.
**Medications:** Ibuprofen.
**PMH:** Headaches at age 20, accompanied by nausea. One episode of sinusitis 4 months ago, treated with amoxicillin.
**PSH:** Tubal ligation 8 years ago.
**SH:** No smoking, no EtOH, no illicit drugs. Patient is an engineer, lives with husband and three children, and is sexually active with husband only.
**FH:** Father died of a brain tumor at age 65. Mother has migraines.

## Physical Examination

Patient is in severe pain.
**VS:** WNL.
**HEENT:** Normocephalic, atraumatic, nontender to palpation, PERRLA, EOMI, no papilledema, no nasal congestion, no pharyngeal erythema or exudates, dentition good.
**Neck:** Supple, no lymphadenopathy.
**Chest:** Clear breath sounds bilaterally.
**Heart:** RRR; normal S1/S2; no murmurs, rubs, or gallops.
**Neuro:** Mental status: Alert and oriented × 3, good concentration. Cranial nerves: 2–12 grossly intact. Motor: Strength 5/5 throughout. DTRs: 2+ intact, symmetric.

## Differential Diagnosis

1. Migraine
2. Tension headache
3. Depression
4. Pseudotumor cerebri
5. Intracranial mass lesion
6. Cluster headache
7. Sinusitis
8. Temporal arteritis

## Diagnostic Workup

1. CBC
2. ESR
3. CT—head or MRI—brain
4. LP
5. CT—sinus
6. Temporal artery biopsy

## CASE DISCUSSION

### Differential Diagnosis

- **Migraine:** Despite lacking an aura, the patient's presentation is classic for this diagnosis.
- **Tension headache:** This is often associated with stress but is usually bilateral and squeezing. It lasts from hours to days and gets worse as the day progresses.
- **Depression:** Headaches may be worse on arising in the morning and are associated with other symptoms of depression.
- **Pseudotumor cerebri:** Headaches can be focal but are usually accompanied by diplopia and other visual symptoms. Exam should reveal papilledema but can be normal during the first few days after onset of illness.
- **Intracranial mass lesion:** One-third of patients with brain tumors present with a primary complaint of headache. Headache is nonspecific and may mimic features of migraine. Certain brain tumors may have a familial basis.
- **Cluster headache:** This involves unilateral periorbital pain, often accompanied by ipsilateral nasal congestion, rhinorrhea, lacrimation, redness of the eye, and/or Horner's syndrome. Episodes of daily pain occur in clusters and often awaken patients at night. However, this occurs rarely in women (a similar entity seen in women is termed *chronic paroxysmal hemicrania*).
- **Sinusitis:** This is a rare cause of headache. There are no signs or symptoms of sinus or respiratory infection in this case.
- **Temporal arteritis:** This affects patients > 50 years of age. Headache is often accompanied by constitutional symptoms, jaw claudication, scalp tenderness, and visual symptoms.

### Diagnostic Workup

- **CBC:** To look for leukocytosis, a nonspecific sign of infection or inflammation. Mild normocytic anemia and thrombocytosis may also be seen in temporal arteritis.
- **ESR:** To screen for evidence of inflammation in suspected temporal arteritis.
- **CT–head or MRI–brain:** Headache syndromes are largely clinical diagnoses. Neuroimaging is generally reserved for patients with acute severe headache, chronic unexplained headache, or abnormalities on neurologic exam. MRI provides greater anatomical detail, but CT is preferred to rule out acute bleeds.
- **LP:** To look for elevated opening pressure in pseudotumor. CSF is otherwise normal. RBCs and xanthochromia can be seen in subarachnoid hemorrhage (perform if suspicion is high despite a negative CT scan).
- **CT–sinus:** To look for sinusitis.
- **Temporal artery biopsy:** Should be performed within one week of starting treatment with high-dose corticosteroids to diagnose temporal arteritis (as noted above, this diagnosis would not be considered in a 35-year-old woman).

# CASE 19

## DOORWAY INFORMATION

### Opening Scenario

Carl Fisher, a 57-year-old male, comes to the ER complaining of bloody urine.

### Vital Signs

**BP:** 130/80 mmHg
**Temp:** 98.5°F (36.9°C)
**RR:** 13/minute
**HR:** 72/minute, regular

### Examinee Tasks

1. Take a focused history.
2. Perform a focused physical exam (do not perform rectal, genitourinary, or female breast exam).
3. Explain your clinical impression and workup plan to the patient.
4. Write the patient note after leaving the room.

### Checklist/SP Sheet

PATIENT DESCRIPTION

Patient is a 57 yo M.

NOTES FOR THE SP

- Show pain when the examinee checks for CVA tenderness on the right.
- If the examinee mentions prostate disease, ask, "What's prostate disease?"

CHALLENGING QUESTIONS TO ASK

"They told me this is because of my old age. Is that true?"

SAMPLE EXAMINEE RESPONSE

"No. Bloody urine is never normal."

### Examinee Checklist

ENTRANCE:

- ☐ Examinee knocked on the door before entering.
- ☐ Examinee introduced self by name.
- ☐ Examinee identified his/her role or position.
- ☐ Examinee correctly used patient's name.
- ☐ Examinee made eye contact with the SP.

HISTORY:

- ☐ Examinee showed compassion for your illness.

| ☑ Question | Patient Response |
|---|---|
| ☐ Chief complaint | I have blood in my urine, doctor. |
| ☐ How did he know it was blood? | It was bright red and later had some clots. |
| ☐ Onset | Yesterday morning. |
| ☐ Progression | That was the only time it has ever happened; my urine is back to normal. |
| ☐ Pain/burning on urination | None. |
| ☐ Fever | None. |
| ☐ Abdominal/flank pain | None. |
| ☐ Polyuria, frequency | Yes. |
| ☐ Straining during urination | Yes. |
| ☐ Nocturia | Yes. |
| ☐ Weak stream | Yes. |
| ☐ Dribbling | Yes. |
| ☐ Onset of the previous symptoms | Two years ago. They told me I am getting old; am I? |
| ☐ History of renal stones | No. |
| ☐ Associated symptoms (nausea/vomiting, diarrhea/constipation) | None. |
| ☐ Constitutional symptoms (weight loss, appetite changes, night sweats) | None. |
| ☐ Previous similar episodes | No. |
| ☐ Current medications | Allopurinol. |
| ☐ Past medical history | Gout. |
| ☐ Past surgical history | Appendectomy at age 23. |
| ☐ Family history | My father died at age 80 because of a kidney problem. My mother is alive and healthy. |
| ☐ Occupation | Painter. |
| ☐ Alcohol use | A couple of beers after work, 2–3 times a week. |
| ☐ Illicit drug use | No. |
| ☐ Tobacco | Yes. |
| ☐ Duration | Thirty years. |
| ☐ Amount | One pack a day. |
| ☐ Sexual activity | I have a new girlfriend; I met her last month in the bar. |
| ☐ Sexual orientation | Women only. |
| ☐ Use of condoms | Sometimes, if they're available. |

| ☑ Question | Patient Response |
|---|---|
| ☐ History of STDs | I have herpes. The last attack was several months ago. The lesions stay for several days and resolve without treatment. |
| ☐ HIV test | Never. |
| ☐ Drug allergies | No. |

## Physical Examination:

☐ Examinee washed his/her hands.
☐ Examinee asked permission to start the exam.
☐ Examinee used respectful draping.
☐ Examinee did not repeat painful maneuvers.

| ☑ Exam Component | Maneuver |
|---|---|
| ☐ CV exam | Auscultation |
| ☐ Pulmonary exam | Auscultation |
| ☐ Abdominal exam | Auscultation, palpation, percussion, checked for CVA tenderness |
| ☐ Extremities | Inspection |

## Closure:

☐ Examinee discussed initial diagnostic impressions.
☐ Examinee discussed initial management plans:
　　☐ Suggested a genital exam.
　　☐ Suggested a rectal exam for the prostate.
　　☐ Diagnostic tests.
☐ Examinee asked if the patient has any other questions or concerns.

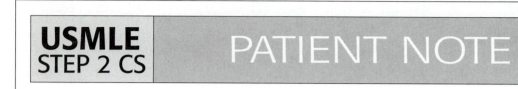

## USMLE STEP 2 CS · PATIENT NOTE

**History**

**Physical Examination**

**Differential Diagnosis**

1.

2.

3.

4.

5.

**Diagnostic Workup**

1.

2.

3.

4.

5.

## History

**HPI:** *57 yo male c/o 1 episode of painless hematuria yesterday morning. He has no fever, no abdominal or flank pain, and no dysuria. No history of renal stones. He has a 2-year history of straining on urination, polyuria, nocturia, weak urinary stream, and dribbling. No nausea, vomiting, diarrhea, or constipation. No change in appetite or weight loss. No previous similar episodes.*
**Allergies:** *NKDA.*
**Medications:** *Allopurinol.*
**PMH:** *Gout; genital herpes that recurred several months ago.*
**PSH:** *Appendectomy, age 23.*
**SH:** *One PPD for 30 years, 2 beers 2–3 times/week, no illicit drugs. Works as a painter. Heterosexual, has a new partner, and uses condoms occasionally.*
**FH:** *Father died at age 80 due to a kidney problem.*

## Physical Examination

*Patient is in no acute distress.*
**VS:** *WNL.*
**Chest:** *Clear breath sounds bilaterally.*
**Heart:** *RRR; normal S1/S2; no murmurs, rubs, or gallops.*
**Abdomen:** *Soft, nondistended, nontender, ⊕BS, no hepatosplenomegaly. Mild right CVA tenderness.*
**Extremities:** *No edema.*

## Differential Diagnosis

1. Bladder cancer
2. Urolithiasis
3. BPH
4. Prostate cancer
5. Renal cell carcinoma
6. Glomerulonephritis
7. UTI

## Diagnostic Workup

1. Genital exam
2. Rectal exam
3. UA
4. Urine culture
5. Urine cytology
6. BUN/Cr
7. PSA
8. U/S—renal/transrectal
9. Cystoscopy
10. CT—abdomen/pelvis
11. IVP

## CASE DISCUSSION

### Differential Diagnosis

A useful mnemonic for the differential diagnosis of hematuria is **HITTERS**—etiologies include **H**ematologic or coagulation disorders, **I**nfection, **T**rauma, **T**umor, **E**xercise, **R**enal disorder, and **S**tones. Gynecologic sources may need to be excluded in women. The passage of clots often localizes the source of bleeding to the lower urinary tract. Gross hematuria in adults represents malignancy until proven otherwise.

- **Bladder cancer:** Hematuria and irritative voiding symptoms are consistent with this diagnosis, and the patient's cigarette smoking and possible occupational exposure to industrial solvents are risk factors. However, the finding of right CVA tenderness is unusual and could be a sign of upper urinary tract disease.
- **Urolithiasis:** Despite the presence of hematuria and CVA tenderness, this very common diagnosis is unlikely in the absence of sudden, severe colicky flank pain. Pain may migrate to the groin and is not alleviated by changes in position.
- **BPH:** The patient's urinary symptoms are classic for this diagnosis except that hematuria (if present) is usually microscopic. Again, CVA tenderness may signal upper urinary tract pathology.
- **Prostate cancer:** As above, this diagnosis is plausible but is hard to reconcile with the presence of CVA tenderness (could postulate metastasis to a right posterior rib).
- **Renal cell carcinoma:** The classic triad is hematuria, flank pain, and a palpable mass. Constitutional symptoms may be prominent. The patient's other urinary symptoms may be due to coexisting BPH.
- **Glomerulonephritis:** The absence of hypertension or signs of volume overload (e.g., edema) argues against intrinsic renal disease. However, remember that IgA nephropathy is the most common acute glomerulonephritis and most commonly presents with an episode of gross hematuria. Presentation is usually concurrent with URI, GI symptoms, or a flulike illness.
- **UTI:** This can cause hematuria but is uncommon in males. The patient has no other symptoms to suggest acute infection.

### Diagnostic Workup

- **Genital exam:** To exclude a gynecologic source of bleeding in women.
- **Rectal exam:** To detect masses as well as prostatic enlargement or nodules.
- **UA:** To assess hematuria, pyuria, bacteriuria, etc. Dysmorphic RBCs or casts are signs of glomerular disease. The absence of hematuria does not rule out urolithiasis.
- **Urine culture:** To exclude UTI.
- **Urine cytology:** Has variable sensitivity in detecting bladder cancers, depending on the tumor's grade and stage. Examine three voided samples to maximize sensitivity.
- **BUN/Cr:** To evaluate kidney function.
- **PSA:** The serum level correlates with the volume of both benign and malignant prostatic tissue. Can be normal in about 20% of patients who have nonmetastatic prostate cancer.
- **U/S—renal/transrectal:** Can detect bladder and renal masses and stones, but is operator dependent and is less sensitive in detecting ureteral disease. Transrectal U/S is used to help stage prostate cancer and to guide prostatic biopsy.
- **Cystoscopy:** The gold standard for the diagnosis of bladder cancer.
- **CT—abdomen/pelvis:** To evaluate the urinary tract. Can identify neoplasms and a variety of benign conditions such as stones.
- **IVP:** Provides an assessment of the kidneys, ureters, and bladder but is generally being replaced by CT—urogram to avoid contrast administration.

## Opening Scenario

James Miller, a 54-year-old male, comes to the clinic for hypertension follow-up.

## Vital Signs

BP: 135/90 mmHg
Temp: 98.0°F (36.7°C)
RR: 16/minute
HR: 70/minute, regular

## Examinee Tasks

1. Obtain a focused history.
2. Perform a focused physical exam (do not perform rectal, genitourinary, or female breast exam).
3. Explain your clinical impression and workup plan to the patient.
4. Write the patient note after leaving the room.

## Checklist/SP Sheet

### PATIENT DESCRIPTION

Patient is a 54 yo M.

### NOTES FOR THE SP

Don't mention impotence unless the examinee asks whether you are having any side effects from your medications or whether you have any other concerns.

### CHALLENGING QUESTIONS TO ASK

"I think it is my age. Isn't that right, doctor?"

### SAMPLE EXAMINEE RESPONSE

"No, I don't think it's because of your age. I worry more about your medications. However, testosterone levels can decrease with age, and we will check for that."

## Examinee Checklist

### ENTRANCE:

☐ Examinee knocked on the door before entering.
☐ Examinee introduced self by name.
☐ Examinee identified his/her role or position.
☐ Examinee correctly used patient's name.
☐ Examinee made eye contact with the SP.

### HISTORY:

☐ Examinee showed compassion for your illness.

| ☑ | Question | Patient Response |
|---|----------|------------------|
| ☐ | Chief complaint | I am here to check on my blood pressure. |
| ☐ | Onset | Last year I found out that I have hypertension. |
| ☐ | Treatment | The doctor started me on hydrochlorothiazide, but my blood pressure stayed high. He added propranolol six months ago. |
| ☐ | Compliance with medications | Well, sometimes I forget to take the pills, but in general I take them regularly. |
| ☐ | Last blood pressure checkup | Six months ago. |
| ☐ | How he is feeling today | Good. |
| ☐ | Home monitoring of blood pressure | No. |
| ☐ | Any other symptoms (fatigue, headaches, dizziness, blurred vision, nausea, palpitations, chest pain, shortness of breath, urinary changes, weakness, bowel movement changes, sleep problems) | No. |
| ☐ | Medication side effects | Over the past four months I started having problems in my sexual performance. A friend told me it is the propranolol, but I think it is my age. Isn't that right, doctor? |
| ☐ | Description of the problem | I have a weak erection. |
| ☐ | Severity on 1–10 scale, where 1 is flaccid and 6 is adequate for penetration | About a 4. |
| ☐ | Early-morning or nocturnal erections | No. |
| ☐ | Libido | That's weak too, doc. I'm just not as interested in sex as I used to be. |
| ☐ | Marital or work problems | No, my wife is great and I am very happy in my job. |
| ☐ | Feelings of depression | No. |
| ☐ | Feelings of anxiety or stress | No. |
| ☐ | Any leg or buttock pain while walking or resting. | No. |
| ☐ | Weight changes | No. |
| ☐ | Appetite changes | No. |
| ☐ | Diabetes | No. |
| ☐ | History of hypercholesterolemia | Yes, it was diagnosed last year. |
| ☐ | Previous heart problems | No. |
| ☐ | History of TIA or stroke | No. |
| ☐ | Current medications | Propranolol, hydrochlorothiazide, lovastatin. |
| ☐ | Past medical history | None. |
| ☐ | Past surgical history | None. |

| ✓ | Question | Patient Response |
|---|----------|------------------|
| ☐ | Family history | My father died at age 50 of a heart attack. My mother is healthy, but she has Alzheimer's disease. She is in a nursing home now. |
| ☐ | Occupation | Schoolteacher. |
| ☐ | Diet | I eat a lot of junk food. |
| ☐ | Exercise | No. |
| ☐ | Alcohol use | Yes, 3–4 beers a week. |
| ☐ | Illicit drug use | No. |
| ☐ | Tobacco | No. |
| ☐ | Social history | I am married and live with my wife. |
| ☐ | Sexual activity | I had a wonderful sex life with my wife until four months ago, when I started having this problem that I told you about. I think I am getting old. |
| ☐ | Drug allergies | No. |

## Physical Examination:

☐ Examinee washed his/her hands.
☐ Examinee asked permission to start the exam.
☐ Examinee used respectful draping.
☐ Examinee did not repeat painful maneuvers.

| ✓ | Exam Component | Maneuver |
|---|----------------|----------|
| ☐ | Head and neck exam | Funduscopic exam, carotid auscultation |
| ☐ | CV exam | Palpation, auscultation |
| ☐ | Pulmonary exam | Auscultation |
| ☐ | Abdominal exam | Auscultation, palpation |
| ☐ | Extremities | Inspection, palpation of peripheral pulses |
| ☐ | Neurologic exam | DTRs, Babinski's sign, sensation and strength in bilateral lower extremities |

## Closure:

☐ Examinee discussed initial diagnostic impressions.
☐ Examinee discussed initial management plans:
    ☐ Follow-up tests: Examinee mentioned the need for genital and rectal exams.
    ☐ Lifestyle modification (diet, exercise, alcohol cessation).
    ☐ Changing propranolol to another antihypertensive medication that does not cause erectile dysfunction.
☐ Examinee asked if the patient has any other questions or concerns.

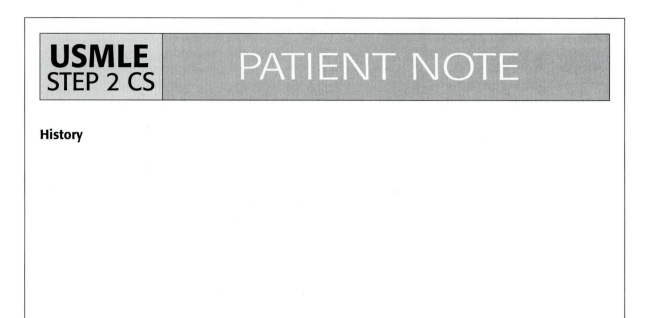

**History**

**Physical Examination**

**Differential Diagnosis**

1.

2.

3.

4.

5.

**Diagnostic Workup**

1.

2.

3.

4.

5.

## History

**HPI:** 54 yo M here for follow-up of his hypertension that was diagnosed last year. He was initially started on HCTZ; propranolol was added 6 months ago. He is fairly compliant with his medications. He does not monitor his blood pressure at home. His last blood pressure checkup was 6 months ago. He is feeling well except for erectile dysfunction and decreased libido noted 4 months ago. No leg claudication or any previous history of heart problems, stroke, TIA, or diabetes. No marital or work problems. No depression, anxiety, appetite or weight changes, or history of trauma.
**ROS:** Negative except for the above.
**Allergies:** NKDA.
**Medications:** HCTZ, propranolol, lovastatin.
**PMH:** Hypertension, hypercholesterolemia diagnosed 1 year ago.
**PSH:** None.
**SH:** No smoking, 3–4 beers/week, no illicit drugs. Works as a schoolteacher; married and lives with his wife.
**FH:** Father died of a heart attack at age 50. Mother is in a nursing home due to Alzheimer's disease.

## Physical Examination

**VS:** WNL.
**HEENT:** No funduscopic abnormalities.
**Neck:** No carotid bruits, no JVD.
**Chest:** Clear breath sounds bilaterally.
**Heart:** Apical impulse not displaced, RRR; S1/S2; no murmurs, rubs, or gallops.
**Abdomen:** Soft, nondistended, nontender, ⊕BS, no bruits, no organomegaly.
**Extremities:** No edema, no hair loss or skin changes. Radial, brachial, femoral, dorsalis pedis, and posterior tibialis 2+ and symmetric.
**Neuro:** Motor: Strength 5/5 in bilateral lower extremities. Sensation: Intact to pinprick and soft touch in lower extremities. DTRs: Symmetric 2+ in lower extremities, ⊖Babinski bilaterally.

## Differential Diagnosis

1. Drug-induced erectile dysfunction (ED)
2. Hypogonadism
3. ED caused by vascular disease
4. Depression
5. Alcohol-related erectile dysfunction
6. Peyronie's disease

## Diagnostic Workup

1. Genital exam
2. Rectal exam
3. Serum glucose
4. Testosterone
5. LH/FSH
6. Prolactin, TSH
7. Ferritin
8. MRI—brain
9. Doppler U/S—penis
10. Dynamic cavernosography
11. BUN/Cr, electrolytes, cholesterol, UA, ECG

## CASE DISCUSSION

### Differential Diagnosis

- **Drug-induced erectile dysfunction (ED):** Antihypertensives (but rarely diuretics), SSRIs, and alcohol are commonly associated with ED. β-blockers may also result in loss of libido.
- **Hypogonadism:** Testosterone deficiency has many underlying etiologies but, as with other endocrine problems, is attributable to either central (due to insufficient gonadotropin secretion by the pituitary) or end-organ disease (pathology in the testes themselves). In addition to diminished libido and possible ED, there are often associated symptoms such as hot flushes, fatigue, and depression.
- **ED caused by vascular disease:** Hypertension and hyperlipidemia are risk factors for atherosclerotic vascular disease, but there are no historical or physical findings (e.g., angina, leg claudication, diminished pulses, hair loss, or thin, shiny skin) to suggest its presence in this case. For example, arterial insufficiency involving the terminal aorta is a common cause of ED but is usually accompanied by vascular claudication of the legs (Leriche's syndrome).
- **Depression:** Psychogenic causes can lead to loss of libido and loss of erections and are suggested when nocturnal or early-morning erections are preserved (not seen in this case). This patient denies other depressive symptoms, but further exploration of his feelings about his demented, nursing-home-bound mother may be more revealing.
- **Alcohol-related ED:** The use of alcohol (as well as tobacco and illicit drugs) is associated with an increased risk of ED.
- **Peyronie's disease:** Fibrous plaque of the tunica albuginea can lead to penile scarring and ED.

### Diagnostic Workup

- **Genital exam:** To rule out Peyronie's disease (e.g., see penile scarring or plaque formation).
- **Rectal exam:** To detect masses or prostatic abnormalities.
- **Serum glucose:** To screen for diabetes, a possible contributor to ED.
- **Testosterone level:** To screen for hypogonadism.
- **LH/FSH:** Gonadotropin levels should be checked in patients with low or borderline testosterone levels. Levels are elevated ("hypergonadotropic") in the setting of testicular pathology and are low ("hypogonadotropic") in the setting of pituitary or hypothalamic disease.
- **Prolactin, TSH:** To screen for other abnormalities of pituitary function in patients with hypogonadotropic hypogonadism.
- **Ferritin:** To screen for hemochromatosis, a common condition; ED can be an early manifestation due to iron deposition in the pituitary gland causing hypogonadotropic hypogonadism.
- **MRI—brain:** To rule out a pituitary or hypothalamic lesion in patients presenting with hypogonadotropic hypogonadism.
- **Doppler U/S—penis:** To assess blood flow in the cavernous arteries.
- **Dynamic cavernosography:** To determine the site and extent of venous leak (suspected in patients with normal arterial inflow).
- **BUN/Cr, electrolytes, cholesterol, UA, ECG:** Useful in the longitudinal care of hypertension and hyperlipidemia. To screen for kidney disease, for LVH or prior silent MIs, for response to cholesterol-lowering medication, and for complications of medical therapy (e.g., diuretic-induced hypokalemia).

# DOORWAY INFORMATION

## Opening Scenario

Kathleen Moore, a 33-year-old female, comes to the clinic complaining of knee pain.

## Vital Signs

BP: 130/80 mmHg
Temp: 99.5°F (37.5°C)
RR: 16/minute
HR: 76/minute, regular

## Examinee Tasks

1. Take a focused history.
2. Perform a focused physical exam (do not perform rectal, genitourinary, or female breast exam).
3. Explain your clinical impression and workup plan to the patient.
4. Write the patient note after leaving the room.

## Checklist/SP Sheet

### PATIENT DESCRIPTION

Patient is a 33 yo F, divorced with two daughters.

### NOTES FOR THE SP

- Pretend to have pain when the examinee moves your left knee in all directions.
- Do not allow the examinee to fully flex or extend your left knee.
- Paint your left knee red to make it look inflamed.

### CHALLENGING QUESTIONS TO ASK

"Do you think I will be able to walk on my knee like before?"

### SAMPLE EXAMINEE RESPONSE

"Most likely yes, but that depends on the underlying problem and your response to treatment."

## Examinee Checklist

### ENTRANCE:

☐ Examinee knocked on the door before entering.
☐ Examinee introduced self by name.
☐ Examinee identified his/her role or position.
☐ Examinee correctly used patient's name.
☐ Examinee made eye contact with the SP.

### HISTORY:

☐ Examinee showed compassion for your pain.

| ☑ *Question* | *Patient Response* |
|---|---|
| ☐ Chief complaint | Left knee pain. |
| ☐ Onset | Two days ago. |
| ☐ Function | I can't move it. I use a cane to walk. |
| ☐ Redness | Yes. |
| ☐ Swelling of the joint | Yes. |
| ☐ Alleviating factors | Rest and Tylenol help a little bit. |
| ☐ Exacerbating factors | Moving my knee and walking. |
| ☐ History of trauma to the knee | No. |
| ☐ Other joint pain | Yes, my wrists and fingers are always painful and stiff. Five years ago I had a painful, swollen big toe on my left foot. |
| ☐ Duration of the pain in the fingers | Six months. |
| ☐ Stiffness in the morning/duration | Yes, for an hour. |
| ☐ Photosensitivity | No. |
| ☐ Rashes | No. |
| ☐ Oral ulcers | I had many in my mouth last month, but they've resolved now. |
| ☐ Fatigue | Yes, I've had no energy to work and have felt tired all the time for the past six months. |
| ☐ Fever/chills | I feel hot now, but I have no chills. |
| ☐ Hair loss | No. |
| ☐ Cold temperature causing problems with the fingers | Sometimes my fingers become pale and then blue when they are exposed to cold weather or cold water. |
| ☐ Heart symptoms (chest pain, palpitations) | No. |
| ☐ Pulmonary complaints (shortness of breath, cough) | No. |
| ☐ Neurologic complaints (seizures, weakness, numbness) | No. |
| ☐ Urinary problems (hematuria) | No. |
| ☐ Abdominal pain | No. |
| ☐ History of recent tick bite | No. |
| ☐ History of pregnancy | I have two daughters. Both were delivered by C-section. |
| ☐ History of abortions/miscarriages | I had two spontaneous abortions a long time ago. |
| ☐ Last menstrual period | Two weeks ago. |
| ☐ Weight changes | I've lost about 10 pounds over the past six months. |
| ☐ Appetite changes | I don't have a good appetite. |

| ☑ Question | Patient Response |
|---|---|
| ☐ Current medications | I used Tylenol to relieve my pain, but it is not working as well anymore. |
| ☐ Past medical history | None. |
| ☐ Past surgical history | Two C-sections at age 23 and 25. |
| ☐ Family history | My mother has rheumatoid arthritis and is living in a nursing home. I don't know my father. |
| ☐ Occupation | Waitress. |
| ☐ Alcohol use | I don't drink a lot, usually 2–4 beers a week except for weekends, when I don't count. |
| ☐ CAGE questions | No (to all four). |
| ☐ Last alcohol ingestion | Four days ago. |
| ☐ Illicit drug use | No. |
| ☐ Tobacco | Yes, one pack a day for the past 20 years. |
| ☐ Sexual activity | I am sexually active with a new boyfriend whom I met two months ago. |
| ☐ Use of condoms | Occasionally. |
| ☐ Number of sexual partners during the last year | Four. |
| ☐ Active with men, women, or both | Men only. |
| ☐ Vaginal discharge | No. |
| ☐ History of sexual transmitted disease | Yes, I had gonorrhea one year ago. I took antibiotics and was fine. |
| ☐ Drug allergies | No. |

## Physical Examination:

☐ Examinee washed his/her hands.
☐ Examinee asked permission to start the exam.
☐ Examinee used respectful draping.
☐ Examinee did not repeat painful maneuvers.

| ☑ Exam Component | Maneuver |
|---|---|
| ☐ Mouth exam | Inspection |
| ☐ Musculoskeletal exam | Inspection and palpation (compared both knees, including range of motion), examined other joints (shoulders, elbows, wrists, hands, fingers, hips, ankles) |
| ☐ Hair and skin exam | Inspection |
| ☐ CV exam | Auscultation |

| ☑ *Exam Component* | *Maneuver* |
|---|---|
| ☐ Pulmonary exam | Auscultation |
| ☐ Abdominal exam | Auscultation, palpation, percussion |

**Closure:**

☐ Examinee discussed initial diagnostic impressions.

☐ Examinee discussed initial management plans:

    ☐ Follow-up tests: Examinee mentioned the need for a pelvic exam.

    ☐ Discussed safe sex practices.

☐ Examinee asked if the patient has any other questions or concerns.

**USMLE**
STEP 2 CS

# PATIENT NOTE

**History**

**Physical Examination**

**Differential Diagnosis**

1.
2.
3.
4.
5.

**Diagnostic Workup**

1.
2.
3.
4.
5.

## History

**HPI:** 33 yo F c/o left knee pain that started 2 days ago and is causing difficulty walking. She has swelling and redness in her left knee and mild fever but no chills. Denies trauma. She has a history of fatigue and painful wrists and fingers and has experienced 1-hour morning stiffness over the past 6 months. She also recalls multiple oral ulcers that resolved last month. Describes Raynaud's phenomenon. She denies rash, photosensitivity, hair loss, or recent tick bites. She recalls a 10-pound weight loss over the past 6 months and has no appetite.
**ROS:** Negative except as above.
**Allergies:** NKDA.
**Medications:** Tylenol.
**PMH:** Episode of acute left big toe arthritis 5 years ago; gonorrhea 1 year ago.
**PSH:** Two C-sections.
**SH:** One PPD for 20 years. Usually drinks 2–4 beers/week; on weekends drinks more, last ingestion 4 days ago, CAGE 0/4. No illicit drugs. Sexually active with multiple partners; inconsistent condom use.
**FH:** Mother has rheumatoid arthritis and lives in a nursing home.

## Physical Examination

**VS:** WNL.
**HEENT:** No oral lesions.
**Chest:** Clear breath sounds bilaterally.
**Heart:** RRR; normal S1/S2; no murmurs, rubs, or gallops.
**Abdomen:** Soft, nondistended, ⊕BS, no hepatosplenomegaly.
**Extremities:** Erythema, tenderness, pain and restricted range of motion on flexion and extension of the left knee compared to the right knee. Shoulder, elbow, wrist, hand, finger, hip, and ankle joints are WNL bilaterally.

## Differential Diagnosis

1. Gout
2. Pseudogout
3. SLE
4. Rheumatoid arthritis
5. Gonococcal septic arthritis
6. Nongonococcal septic arthritis
7. Osteoarthritis

## Diagnostic Workup

1. Pelvic exam and cervical cultures
2. Knee aspiration and synovial fluid analysis
3. CBC
4. Blood culture
5. UA
6. ANA, anti-dsDNA, RF
7. XR—left knee and both hands
8. Serum uric acid

# CASE DISCUSSION

## Differential Diagnosis

- **Gout:** This acute, usually monarticular, crystal-induced arthritis rarely occurs in premenopausal women, but the patient's history of first MTP arthritis ("podagra") is classic for gout. Alcohol ingestion causes hyperuricemia and may precipitate an acute attack. Foot, ankle, and knee joints are also commonly affected. Gout does not explain her hand arthralgias, but osteoarthritis is common and may coexist.

- **Pseudogout:** Another crystal-induced arthritis, pseudogout frequently involves the knees and wrists but is usually seen in patients > 60 years of age.

- **SLE:** Joint symptoms (usually symmetric peripheral arthralgias), constitutional symptoms, and Raynaud's phenomenon may be early manifestations of this disease. Unilateral knee involvement is not typical. The diagnosis requires at least four of the following 11 criteria: malar ("butterfly") rash, discoid rash, symmetric arthritis, photosensitivity, oral ulcers, serositis, renal disease, CNS involvement, hematologic disorders (her fatigue may be due to anemia), immunologic abnormalities (her history of spontaneous abortions may signal the presence of antiphospholipid antibodies), or ANA positivity. More testing needs to be done before SLE can be diagnosed in this case.

- **Rheumatoid arthritis:** This is suggested in a patient with a positive family history, symmetric small joint arthritis (e.g., fingers, wrists), prolonged morning stiffness, and systemic symptoms (low-grade fever, anorexia, weight loss, fatigue, and weakness). However, this patient's hand joints were not red, warm, swollen, or tender on exam. Monarthritis is also uncommon but is occasionally seen early in the course of disease.

- **Gonococcal septic arthritis:** This occurs in healthy hosts, most commonly young women (women are much more likely than men to have asymptomatic genitourinary gonococcal infection, which allows the bug to mutate and disseminate). The knee is the most frequently involved joint, but the monarthritis (or tenosynovitis) is usually preceded by a few days of migratory polyarthralgias. Also, this patient does not have the characteristic rash, which consists of small necrotic pustules on the extremities (including the palms and soles).

- **Nongonococcal septic arthritis:** This occurs suddenly, usually affects the knee or wrist, and is most commonly caused by *S. aureus*. However, it is a disease of an abnormal host; previous joint damage and IVDU are key risk factors not present in this case.

- **Osteoarthritis:** Onset is insidious, joint stiffness brief, and joint inflammation minimal, all of which are incongruent with this patient's presentation. Also, osteoarthritis spares the wrist and MCP joints and is not associated with constitutional symptoms.

## Diagnostic Workup

- **Pelvic exam and cervical cultures:** Necessary to investigate gonococcal infection and are often positive in the absence of symptoms (urine, anorectal, and throat cultures may also be necessary).

- **Knee aspiration, Gram stain, culture, and inspection for crystals:** In most cases of acute monarthritis, joint aspiration must be performed to rule out septic arthritis. Inflammatory joint synovial fluid contains > 3000 WBCs/μL, and septic joint fluid often contains > 50,000 cells/μL. The demonstration of needle-shaped, negatively birefringent crystals or rhomboid-shaped, weakly positively birefringent crystals confirms gout or pseudogout, respectively.

- **CBC:** Look for anemia, leukopenia, and/or thrombocytopenia in SLE, or leukocytosis in acute gout and septic arthritis.

- **Blood culture:** An important test in septic arthritis.

- **UA:** Look for proteinuria, hematuria, and cellular casts in SLE.

- **Immunologic tests:** **ANA** is a highly sensitive (but nonspecific) screening test for SLE. A negative test essentially excludes the disease. If ANA is positive, investigate antibody against double-stranded DNA (**anti-dsDNA**), antibody against the Smith antigen, anticardiolipin antibodies, and lupus anticoagulant to help confirm SLE. **RF** is present in > 75% of patients with rheumatoid arthritis.

- **XR—left knee and both hands:** Specific changes in rheumatoid arthritis include symmetric joint space narrowing, marginal bony erosions, and periarticular demineralization. However, x-rays are usually normal during the first six months of illness. In gout, look for punched-out cortical erosions and a sclerotic joint margin. In pseudogout, look for calcified articular cartilage ("chondrocalcinosis"). In osteoarthritis, look for joint space narrowing, marginal osteophytes, subchondral osteosclerosis, and occasionally subchondral cysts.

- **Serum uric acid:** Has limited diagnostic value because of the frequency of hyperuricemia in the absence of gout. Also, although serum uric acid is almost always elevated in gout, it may be normal during an acute attack (due to spontaneous variation).

## Opening Scenario

Charles Andrews, a 66-year-old male, comes to the clinic complaining of a tremor.

## Vital Signs

**BP:** 135/90 mmHg
**Temp:** 98.6°F (37°C)
**RR:** 16/minute
**HR:** 70/minute, regular

## Examinee Tasks

1. Take a focused history.
2. Perform a focused physical exam (do not perform rectal, genitourinary, or female breast exam).
3. Explain your clinical impression and workup plan to the patient.
4. Write the patient note after leaving the room.

## Checklist/SP Sheet

### PATIENT DESCRIPTION
Patient is a 66 yo M.

### NOTES FOR THE SP

- Exhibit mild muscle rigidity in your wrists and arms—that is, when the examinee tries to move your wrists and arms, stiffen them and move them slowly.
- Lean your back forward slightly and walk in small, shuffling steps.
- Exhibit a resting hand tremor (pill rolling) that disappears with movement.

### CHALLENGING QUESTIONS TO ASK
"Do you think I will get better?"

### SAMPLE EXAMINEE RESPONSE
"I think your tremor will improve with medication, but I don't know how long the improvement will last. The tremor may be a sign of a larger movement disorder called Parkinson's disease, and we need to do more evaluation to explore that possibility."

## Examinee Checklist

### ENTRANCE:

- ☐ Examinee knocked on the door before entering.
- ☐ Examinee introduced self by name.
- ☐ Examinee identified his/her role or position.

☐ Examinee correctly used patient's name.

☐ Examinee made eye contact with the SP.

## HISTORY:

☐ Examinee showed compassion for your illness.

| ☑ Question | Patient Response |
|---|---|
| ☐ Chief complaint | I have a tremor in this hand (points to right hand). |
| ☐ Location | Only in the right hand. |
| ☐ Duration | I noticed it about six months ago, but it seems to be getting worse recently. |
| ☐ Context | It shakes when I'm just sitting around doing nothing. It usually stops when I hold out the remote control to change the channel. |
| ☐ Alleviating factors | None. |
| ☐ Exacerbating factors | It seems more severe when I am really tired. |
| ☐ Associated symptoms (falls, headaches, TIA symptoms, drooling, changes in voice or handwriting, difficulty with ADLs/IADLs, depression, constipation, rash, etc.) | No, I don't think so. My wife says I've slowed down, but I think that's just because I retired last year. (If asked what your wife means, say that she is frustrated because it is your job to push the grocery cart, but you can't keep up with her in the store anymore.) |
| ☐ Prior history of similar symptoms | Well, back in college I occasionally had a hand tremor after pulling an all-nighter and drinking lots of coffee. The tremor was in both hands, but it was worse in the right. It seemed faster than the one I have now. |
| ☐ Caffeine intake | One cup of coffee every morning. I used to drink three cups a day, but I've cut back over the past few months. |
| ☐ Alcohol use | None. Both of my parents were alcoholics, so I never touch it. |
| ☐ Past medical history | High cholesterol, treated with diet. Asthma, treated with an albuterol inhaler as needed. |
| ☐ History of head trauma | No. |
| ☐ Family history | My parents died in a car accident in their 40s, and my sister is healthy. |
| ☐ Social history | I am married and live with my wife. |
| ☐ Occupation | Retired chemistry professor. |
| ☐ Exercise | No, I'm really not very active anymore. |
| ☐ Tobacco | No. |
| ☐ Illicit drug use | No. |
| ☐ Medications | Albuterol inhaler as needed. (If asked, say that you have not used it in more than a year.) |
| ☐ Drug allergies | No. |

**Physical Examination:**

- ☐ Examinee washed his/her hands.
- ☐ Examinee asked permission to start the exam.
- ☐ Examinee used respectful draping.
- ☐ Examinee did not repeat painful maneuvers.

| ☑ *Exam Component* | *Maneuver* |
| --- | --- |
| ☐ CV exam | Auscultation |
| ☐ Pulmonary exam | Auscultation |
| ☐ Neurologic exam | Mental status, cranial nerves, motor (including muscle tone), DTRs, cerebellar, gait, sensory |

**Closure:**

- ☐ Examinee discussed initial diagnostic impressions.
- ☐ Examinee discussed initial management plans:
  - ☐ Follow-up tests.
  - ☐ Discussed possible need to compare an old handwriting sample with a present sample.
  - ☐ Physician support throughout the patient's illness.
- ☐ Examinee asked if the patient has any other questions or concerns.

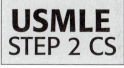

**USMLE STEP 2 CS**

## PATIENT NOTE

**History**

**Physical Examination**

**Differential Diagnosis**

1.

2.

3.

4.

5.

**Diagnostic Workup**

1.

2.

3.

4.

5.

## History

**HPI:** *66 yo M c/o right hand tremor for 6 months. It occurs at rest and seems to be getting worse recently. The tremor is exacerbated by fatigue, and there are no alleviating factors (he does not drink alcohol). Reducing his caffeine intake to 1 cup of coffee daily did not seem to help. He denies associated symptoms but does say that his wife complains that he has "slowed down" since retiring last year. Specifically, he seems to be walking more slowly recently (time course unspecified, but within the past year). He had a hand tremor when very fatigued back in college, but it was bilateral and faster than his present tremor.*
**ROS:** *Negative except as above.*
**Allergies:** *NKDA.*
**Medications:** *Albuterol MDI prn (no use in past year).*
**PMH:** *High cholesterol, treated with diet. Mild asthma.*
**SH:** *No smoking, no EtOH, no illicit drugs. He is a retired chemistry professor, married and lives with his wife.*
**FH:** *Noncontributory.*

## Physical Examination

*Patient is in no acute distress.*
**VS:** *WNL.*
**Chest:** *Clear breath sounds bilaterally.*
**Heart:** *RRR; normal S1/S2; no murmurs, rubs, or gallops.*
**Neuro:** *Alert and oriented × 3. Cranial nerves: 2–12 grossly intact. Motor: Right hand resting tremor, about 6 Hz, "pill rolling," improves or disappears during purposeful action or posture. Mild muscle rigidity in both wrists and arms, but no frank cogwheeling. Strength 5/5 throughout. DTRs: Symmetric 2+ in all extremities. Cerebellar: ⊖Romberg, rapid alternating movements and heel-to-shin test normal and symmetric. Gait: Brady-kinetic, takes small steps. Walks with back slightly bent forward. Sensory: Intact to soft touch and pinprick.*

## Differential Diagnosis

1. Parkinson's disease
2. Essential tremor
3. Physiologic tremor
4. Midbrain lesion
5. Drug-induced tremor
6. Psychogenic tremor
7. Wilson's disease

## Diagnostic Workup

1. TSH
2. Heavy metal screen
3. MRI—brain
4. Ceruloplasmin, slit lamp examination for Kayser-Fleischer rings, AST/ALT, CBC, 24-hour urinary copper, liver biopsy

## CASE DISCUSSION

### Differential Diagnosis

- **Parkinson's disease (PD):** This is the most common cause of resting tremor (i.e., it is evident with the affected body part supported and completely at rest but improves or subsides with voluntary activity), although some patients with PD also have a postural-action tremor that is indistinguishable from essential tremor (ET, see below). Tremor is usually low frequency (4–6 Hz), begins in one upper extremity, and may later involve the other extremities as well. Leg tremor is more commonly due to PD than to ET. The face, lips, and jaw may be involved, but in contrast to ET, PD does not produce head tremor. Along with the tremor, the patient's bradykinesia and rigidity suggest PD.
- **Essential tremor (ET):** This is the most common neurologic cause of postural tremor (i.e., tremor that is apparent when the arms are held outstretched) or action tremor (i.e., tremor that increases at the end of goal-directed activity such as finger-to-nose testing). Approximately 50% of cases are familial. Tremor is usually high frequency and often asymmetrically involves the distal upper extremity. The head, voice, chin, trunk, and legs can also be involved. ET is not associated with other neurologic signs and is improved following the ingestion of small amounts of alcohol. Differentiation from the classical resting tremor of PD is usually straightforward, as in this case.
- **Physiologic tremor:** This refers to very low-amplitude, high-frequency (10–12 Hz) tremor present in normal individuals. The tremor is often not visible, but when enhanced by medications or other medical conditions, it is the most common cause of postural and action tremors. Conditions that can enhance physiologic tremor include anxiety, excitement, sleep deprivation/fatigue, hypoglycemia, caffeine intake, alcohol withdrawal, thyrotoxicosis, fever, and pheochromocytoma.
- **Midbrain lesion:** Midbrain injury due to stroke, trauma, or demyelinating disease is a rare cause of a solitary asymmetric resting tremor.
- **Drug-induced tremor:** Many medications can enhance physiologic tremor, notably β-agonists (such as albuterol), nicotine, theophylline, TCAs, lithium, valproic acid, and corticosteroids. Mercury and arsenic exposure may also contribute to tremor. Neuroleptics and metoclopramide can cause drug-induced parkinsonism, but tremor is often absent in these cases.
- **Psychogenic tremor:** This often manifests with varying frequency and either becomes more irregular or subsides entirely when the patient is asked to perform a complex, repetitive motor task with the contralateral limb.
- **Wilson's disease:** This can cause resting tremor (among other manifestations) but is not considered in patients > 40 years of age.

### Diagnostic Workup

- **TSH:** To screen for hyperthyroidism.
- **Heavy metal screen:** To screen for mercury and arsenic toxicity via urine or blood tests.
- **MRI–brain:** To rule out a structural lesion, particularly in the midbrain or basal ganglia.
- **Ceruloplasmin, slit lamp examination for Kayser-Fleischer rings, AST/ALT, CBC, 24-hour urinary copper, liver biopsy:** These tests comprise the screening tests (and diagnostic tests, in the case of liver biopsy) used to evaluate for suspected Wilson's disease. As noted above, the patient's advanced age precludes consideration of Wilson's disease in this case.

# CASE 23

## DOORWAY INFORMATION

### Opening Scenario

Jay Keller, a 49-year-old male, comes to the ER complaining of passing out a few hours earlier.

### Vital Signs

**BP:** 135/90 mmHg
**Temp:** 98.0°F (36.7°C)
**RR:** 16/minute
**HR:** 76/minute, regular

### Examinee Tasks

1. Take a focused history.
2. Perform a focused physical exam (do not perform rectal, genitourinary, or female breast exam).
3. Explain your clinical impression and workup plan to the patient.
4. Write the patient note after leaving the room.

### Checklist/SP Sheet

PATIENT DESCRIPTION

49 yo M, married with three children.

NOTES FOR THE SP

None.

CHALLENGING QUESTIONS TO ASK

"Do you think I have a brain tumor?"

SAMPLE EXAMINEE RESPONSE

"I think it's unlikely. To make absolutely sure, however, we will do a 'CAT' scan, which is a special x-ray test of the brain. That will help us to see the structure of the brain and to rule out any bleeding or tumor."

### Examinee Checklist

ENTRANCE:

- ☐ Examinee knocked on the door before entering.
- ☐ Examinee introduced self by name.
- ☐ Examinee identified his/her role or position.
- ☐ Examinee correctly used patient's name.
- ☐ Examinee made eye contact with the SP.

HISTORY:

- ☐ Examinee showed compassion for your illness.

| ☑ **Question** | **Patient Response** |
|---|---|
| ☐ Chief complaint | I passed out. |
| ☐ Describe what happened | This morning I was taking the groceries to the car with my wife when I suddenly fell down and blacked out. |
| ☐ Loss of consciousness before, during, or after the fall | I think I lost consciousness and then fell down on the ground. |
| ☐ Duration of loss of consciousness | My wife told me that I did not respond to her for several minutes. |
| ☐ Palpitations before the fall | Yes, just before I fell down, my heart started racing. |
| ☐ Sensing something unusual before losing consciousness (sounds, lights, smells, etc.) | No. |
| ☐ Spinning/lightheadedness | I felt lightheaded right before the fall. |
| ☐ Shaking (seizure) | Yes, my wife told me that my arms and legs started shaking after I fell down. |
| ☐ Duration of shaking | Maybe 30 seconds. |
| ☐ Bit tongue | No. |
| ☐ Lost control of the bladder | No. |
| ☐ Weakness/numbness | No. |
| ☐ Speech difficulties | No. |
| ☐ Confusion after regaining consciousness | No. |
| ☐ Headaches | No. |
| ☐ Chest pain, shortness of breath | No. |
| ☐ Abdominal pain, nausea/vomiting, diarrhea/constipation | No. |
| ☐ Head trauma | No. |
| ☐ Similar falls, lightheadedness, or passing out before | No. |
| ☐ Gait abnormality | No. |
| ☐ Weight changes | No. |
| ☐ Appetite changes | No. |
| ☐ Current medications | Hydrochlorothiazide, captopril, aspirin, atenolol. |
| ☐ Past medical history | High blood pressure for the last 15 years; heart attack one year ago. |
| ☐ Past surgical history | Appendectomy. |
| ☐ Family history | My father died from a heart attack at age 55, and my mother died in good health. |

| ☑ *Question* | *Patient Response* |
|---|---|
| ☐ Occupation | Clerk in a video store. |
| ☐ Alcohol use | Yes, I drink 3–4 beers a week. |
| ☐ CAGE questions | No (to all four). |
| ☐ Illicit drug use | No. |
| ☐ Tobacco | No, I stopped a year ago. I had smoked one pack a day for the previous 25 years. |
| ☐ Sexual activity | Yes, with my wife. |
| ☐ Drug allergies | No. |

## Physical Examination:

☐ Examinee washed his/her hands.

☐ Examinee asked permission to start the exam.

☐ Examinee used respectful draping.

☐ Examinee did not repeat painful maneuvers.

| ☑ *Exam Component* | *Maneuver* |
|---|---|
| ☐ Head and neck exam | Inspection (head, mouth), carotid auscultation and palpation, thyroid exam |
| ☐ CV exam | Palpation, auscultation, orthostatic VS |
| ☐ Pulmonary exam | Auscultation |
| ☐ Extremities | Palpate peripheral pulses |
| ☐ Neurologic exam | Mental status, cranial nerves (including funduscopic exam), motor, DTRs, cerebellar, Romberg test, gait, sensory |

## Closure:

☐ Examinee discussed initial diagnostic impressions.

☐ Examinee discussed initial management plans:

    ☐ Follow-up tests.

☐ Examinee asked if the patient has any other questions or concerns.

USMLE STEP 2 CS

# PATIENT NOTE

**History**

**Physical Examination**

**Differential Diagnosis**

1.
2.
3.
4.
5.

**Diagnostic Workup**

1.
2.
3.
4.
5.

## History

**HPI:** 49 yo M c/o 1 episode of syncope that occurred a few hours ago. He was taking the groceries to the car with his wife when he suddenly felt lightheaded, had palpitations, lost consciousness, and fell down. He was unconscious for several minutes. His wife recalls that his arms and legs started shaking for 30 seconds after he fell down. He denies subsequent confusion, weakness or numbness, speech difficulties, tongue biting, or incontinence.
**ROS:** Negative except as above.
**Allergies:** NKDA.
**Medications:** HCTZ, captopril, aspirin, atenolol.
**PMH:** Hypertension for the last 15 years; MI 1 year ago.
**PSH:** Appendectomy.
**SH:** One PPD for 25 years; quit 1 year ago. Drinks 2–3 beers/week, CAGE 0/4, no illicit drugs.
**FH:** Father died from an MI at age 55.

## Physical Examination

**VS:** WNL, no orthostatic changes.
**HEENT:** Normocephalic, atraumatic, PERRLA, no funduscopic abnormalities, no tongue trauma.
**Neck:** Supple, no carotid bruits, 2+ carotid pulses with good upstroke bilaterally, thyroid normal.
**Chest:** Clear breath sounds bilaterally.
**Heart:** Apical impulse not displaced; RRR; normal S1/S2; no murmurs, rubs, or gallops.
**Extremities:** Symmetric 2+ brachial, radial, and dorsalis pedis pulses bilaterally.
**Neuro:** Cranial nerves: 2–12 grossly intact. Motor: Strength 5/5 throughout. Sensation: Intact to pinprick and soft touch bilaterally. DTRs: Symmetric 2+ in upper and lower extremities, ⊖Babinski bilaterally. Cerebellar: Romberg, finger to nose normal. Gait: Normal.

## Differential Diagnosis

1. Convulsive syncope
2. Vasovagal syncope
3. Cardiac arrhythmia
4. Aortic stenosis
5. Drug-induced orthostatic hypotension
6. Seizure

## Diagnostic Workup

1. CBC, electrolytes
2. CXR
3. CT—head or MRI—brain
4. ECG and Holter monitor
5. Echocardiography
6. Doppler U/S—carotid
7. Prolactin
8. EEG

## CASE DISCUSSION

### Differential Diagnosis

- **Convulsive syncope:** Seizure-like activity often occurs after syncope and is due to global cerebral hypoperfusion. There is no EEG correlate, and a seizure workup is not required.
- **Vasovagal syncope:** This often occurs in the setting of emotional stress or pain and may be due to excessive vagal tone with resulting hypotension. Syncope is often heralded by nausea, sweating, tachycardia, pallor, and feeling "faint." This is also the mechanism of syncope in postmicturition syncope.
- **Cardiac arrhythmia:** Cardiac syncope typically occurs without warning, although a history of palpitations may indicate the presence of an underlying arrhythmia. This patient's history of MI increases his risk of developing ventricular tachycardia, and β-blocker therapy may contribute to bradyarrhythmia.
- **Aortic stenosis:** This and other mechanical causes (e.g., hypertrophic obstructive cardiomyopathy, atrial myxoma) are commonly exertional or postexertional and occur without warning. The lack of a murmur and other physical findings makes this unlikely in this case.
- **Drug-induced orthostatic hypotension:** The patient's antihypertensive medications increase his risk for orthostatic hypotension and syncope. However, lightheadedness and syncope in this condition is usually postural (i.e., occurs when getting up from a lying or seated position), and this patient's orthostatic vital signs were normal.
- **Seizure:** Seizures usually occur unpredictably in a manner unrelated to posture or exertion. They may stem from a variety of causes, including metabolic factors, trauma, vascular factors, and brain tumors. Tonic-clonic seizures are often accompanied by tongue biting, incontinence, and prolonged confusion or drowsiness postictally.

### Diagnostic Workup

- **CBC, electrolytes:** To rule out anemia, evidence of hyperviscosity, or electrolyte imbalance that could lead to arrhythmia or other causes of syncope.
- **CXR:** To rule out lung mass, cardiomyopathy, or other pathology.
- **CT–head:** The test of choice to exclude intracranial hemorrhage. Also rules out tumor, trauma, prior stroke, or abscess.
- **MRI–brain:** Provides better anatomical detail than CT. Indicated when focal neurologic signs and symptoms are present. MRA is helpful when vertebrobasilar insufficiency is suspected (i.e., when syncope is accompanied by other brain stem signs).
- **ECG and Holter or event monitor:** To evaluate possible arrhythmia.
- **Echocardiography:** To rule out mechanical causes of syncope (e.g., severe aortic stenosis, atrial myxoma, severe LVH with small residual cavity size, and hypertrophic obstructive cardiomyopathy).
- **Doppler U/S–carotid:** To exclude bilateral carotid stenosis.
- **Prolactin:** Often elevated within 30–60 minutes following a generalized seizure (it is useless after that time interval). Must be compared to baseline prolactin levels.
- **EEG:** To evaluate suspected seizure activity.

# CASE 24
## DOORWAY INFORMATION

### Opening Scenario

Kristin Grant, a 30-year-old female, comes to the office complaining of weight gain.

### Vital Signs

BP: 120/85 mmHg
Temp: 98.0°F (36.7°C)
RR: 13/minute
HR: 65/minute, regular
BMI: 30

### Examinee Tasks

1. Take a focused history.
2. Perform a focused physical exam (do not perform rectal, genitourinary, or female breast exam).
3. Explain your clinical impression and workup plan to the patient.
4. Write the patient note after leaving the room.

### Checklist/SP Sheet

PATIENT DESCRIPTION
Patient is a 30 yo F.

NOTES FOR THE SP
None.

CHALLENGING QUESTIONS TO ASK
"I want to go back to smoking because I believe that I have started gaining weight since I quit."

SAMPLE EXAMINEE RESPONSE
"I understand that your weight is very important to you, but it's clear that the health consequences of smoking far outweigh those associated with weight gain. We also need to determine what else might be contributing to your weight gain and then discuss strategies to deal with it."

### Examinee Checklist

ENTRANCE:

- ☐ Examinee knocked on the door before entering.
- ☐ Examinee introduced self by name.
- ☐ Examinee identified his/her role or position.
- ☐ Examinee correctly used patient's name.
- ☐ Examinee made eye contact with the SP.

## HISTORY:

☐ Examinee showed compassion for your illness.

| ☑ Question | Patient Response |
|---|---|
| ☐ Chief complaint | I am gaining weight. |
| ☐ Onset | Three months ago. |
| ☐ Pounds gained | Twenty pounds. |
| ☐ Cold intolerance | Yes. |
| ☐ Skin/hair changes | My hair is falling out more than usual, and I feel that my skin has become dry. |
| ☐ Voice change | No. |
| ☐ Constipation | No. |
| ☐ Appetite changes | I have a good appetite. |
| ☐ Fatigue | No. |
| ☐ Depression | No. |
| ☐ Sleeping problems (falling asleep, staying asleep, early waking, snoring) | No. |
| ☐ Associated symptoms (fever/chills, chest pain, shortness of breath, abdominal pain, diarrhea) | No. |
| ☐ Last menstrual period | One week ago. |
| ☐ Frequency of menstrual periods | I used to get my period every four weeks, but recently I've been getting it every six weeks or more. The period lasts seven days. |
| ☐ Start of change in cycle | Six months ago. |
| ☐ Pads/tampons changed a day | It was 2–3 a day, but the blood flow is becoming less, and I use only one a day now. |
| ☐ Age at menarche | Age 13. |
| ☐ Pregnancies | I have one child; he is 10 years old. |
| ☐ Problems during pregnancy/delivery | No, it was a normal delivery, and my child is healthy. |
| ☐ Miscarriages/abortions | None. |
| ☐ Hirsutism | No. |
| ☐ Current medications | Lithium. |
| ☐ Past medical history | I have bipolar disorder. I was started on lithium six months ago; I haven't had any problems since then. |
| ☐ Past surgical history | None. |
| ☐ Family history of obesity | My mother and sister are obese. |
| ☐ Occupation | Housekeeper. |

| ☑ Question | Patient Response |
|---|---|
| ☐ Alcohol use | None. |
| ☐ Illicit drug use | Never. |
| ☐ Tobacco | I quit smoking three months ago. I had smoked two packs a day for 10 years. |
| ☐ Exercise | No. |
| ☐ Diet | The usual. I haven't changed anything in my diet in more than 10 years. Donuts, lots of coffee during the day, chicken, steak, Chinese food, and salad. |
| ☐ Sexual activity | With my husband. |
| ☐ Contraceptives | My husband had a vasectomy two years ago. |
| ☐ Drug allergies | No. |

## Physical Examination:

☐ Examinee washed his/her hands.
☐ Examinee asked permission to start the exam.
☐ Examinee used respectful draping.
☐ Examinee did not repeat painful maneuvers.

| ☑ Exam Component | Maneuver |
|---|---|
| ☐ Head exam | Inspected conjunctivae, mouth, and throat |
| ☐ Neck exam | Palpated lymph nodes, thyroid gland |
| ☐ CV exam | Auscultation |
| ☐ Pulmonary exam | Auscultation |
| ☐ Abdominal exam | Auscultation, percussion, palpation |
| ☐ Extremities | Inspection, checked DTRs |

## Closure:

☐ Examinee discussed initial diagnostic impressions.
☐ Examinee discussed initial management plans:
  ☐ Diagnostic tests.
  ☐ Lifestyle modification (diet, exercise, relaxation techniques, smoking cessation support).
☐ Examinee asked if the patient has any other questions or concerns.

# PATIENT NOTE

**History**

**Physical Examination**

| **Differential Diagnosis** | **Diagnostic Workup** |
|---|---|
| 1. | 1. |
| 2. | 2. |
| 3. | 3. |
| 4. | 4. |
| 5. | 5. |

# PATIENT NOTE

## History

**HPI:** 30 yo F c/o weight gain of 20 pounds over the past 3 months after she stopped smoking. She has a good appetite and reports no change in her diet. For 6 months she has experienced oligomenorrhea and hypomenorrhea, dry skin, and cold intolerance. No voice change, no constipation, no hirsutism, no depression, no fatigue, and no sleep problems.

**OB/GYN:** Last menstrual period last week. See HPI for other.

**ROS:** Negative except as above.

**Allergies:** NKDA.

**Medications:** Lithium, started 6 months ago.

**PMH:** Bipolar disorder, diagnosed 6 months ago.

**SH:** Two PPD for 10 years; stopped 3 months ago. No alcohol, no illicit drugs. Sexually active with husband only. Doesn't exercise.

**Diet:** Consists mainly of donuts, lots of coffee during the day, chicken, steak, Chinese food, and salad.

**FH:** Mother and sister are obese.

## Physical Examination

Patient is in no acute distress.

**VS:** WNL.

**HEENT:** No conjunctival pallor, mouth and pharynx WNL.

**Neck:** No lymphadenopathy, thyroid normal.

**Chest:** Clear breath sounds bilaterally.

**Heart:** RRR; normal S1/S2; no murmurs, rubs, or gallops.

**Abdomen:** Soft, nontender, nondistended, $\oplus$BS, no hepatosplenomegaly.

**Extremities:** No edema, normal DTRs in lower extremities bilaterally.

## Differential Diagnosis

1. Smoking cessation
2. Hypothyroidism
3. Lithium-related obesity
4. Familial obesity
5. Pregnancy
6. Cushing's syndrome

## Diagnostic Workup

1. TSH
2. Urine hCG
3. Glucose, cholesterol, triglycerides
4. Dexamethasone suppression test
5. 24-hour urine free cortisol

## CASE DISCUSSION

### Differential Diagnosis

- **Smoking cessation:** Weight gain occurs in most patients following smoking cessation but usually averages only 2 kg (4.4 lbs). However, major weight gain such as that seen in this case may occur. Patients generally report increased appetite and calorie consumption.
- **Hypothyroidism:** The patient has classic symptoms of hypothyroidism, and it needs to be ruled out as a cause of her weight gain.
- **Lithium-related obesity:** Weight gain is a common side effect of lithium therapy and may contribute in this case.
- **Familial obesity:** There are probably strong genetic influences on the development of obesity, but a positive family history does not account for acute weight gain.
- **Pregnancy:** Regardless of the menstrual history given by the patient, suspect pregnancy in a woman of childbearing age who has unexplained weight gain.
- **Cushing's syndrome:** This is a rare cause of unexplained weight gain and can usually be diagnosed by physical exam (e.g., one can see hypertension, moon facies, plethora, supraclavicular fat pads, truncal obesity with thin limbs, and abdominal striae).

### Diagnostic Workup

- **TSH:** To diagnose suspected hypothyroidism.
- **Urine hCG:** To rule out pregnancy.
- **Glucose, cholesterol, triglycerides:** To screen for medical complications of obesity.
- **Dexamethasone suppression test:** To screen for hypercortisolism. A suppressed morning cortisol following bedtime dexamethasone administration excludes Cushing's syndrome with 98% certainty.
- **24-hour urine free cortisol:** Performed if the dexamethasone suppression test is abnormal. Helps confirm hypercortisolism.

# CASE 25

## DOORWAY INFORMATION

### Opening Scenario

Patricia Garrison, a 36-year-old female, comes to the office complaining of not having menstrual periods recently.

### Vital Signs

**BP:** 120/85 mmHg
**Temp:** 98.0°F (36.7°C)
**RR:** 13/minute
**HR:** 65/minute, regular

### Examinee Tasks

1. Take a focused history.
2. Perform a focused physical exam (do not perform rectal, genitourinary, or female breast exam).
3. Explain your clinical impression and workup plan to the patient.
4. Write the patient note after leaving the room.

### Checklist/SP Sheet

PATIENT DESCRIPTION

Patient is a 36 yo F.

NOTES FOR THE SP

None.

CHALLENGING QUESTIONS TO ASK

"Am I going through menopause?"

SAMPLE EXAMINEE RESPONSE

"I doubt it. It would be extremely unusual at your age. I need to learn more by asking you about other symptoms and examining you, and then we can discuss possible reasons you are not having periods."

### Examinee Checklist

ENTRANCE:

- ☐ Examinee knocked on the door before entering.
- ☐ Examinee introduced self by name.
- ☐ Examinee identified his/her role or position.
- ☐ Examine correctly used patient's name.
- ☐ Examinee made eye contact with the SP.

☐    Examinee showed compassion for your illness.

| ☑ Question | Patient Response |
|---|---|
| ☐ Chief complaint | I haven't had a period in three months. |
| ☐ Menstrual history | I used to have regular periods every month lasting for 4–5 days, but over the last year I started having them less frequently—every 5–6 weeks lasting for seven days. |
| ☐ Pads/tampons changed a day | It was 2–3 a day, but the blood flow is becoming less, and I use only one a day now. |
| ☐ Age at menarche | Age 14. |
| ☐ Weight change | I have gained 15 pounds over the past year. |
| ☐ Cold intolerance | No. |
| ☐ Skin/hair changes | Actually, I noticed some facial hair recently that I am plucking. |
| ☐ Voice change | No. |
| ☐ Change in bowel habits | No. |
| ☐ Appetite changes | I have a good appetite. |
| ☐ Fad diet or diet pills | No, I've been a vegetarian for 10 years. |
| ☐ Fatigue | No. |
| ☐ Depression/anxiety/stress | No. |
| ☐ Hot flushes | No. |
| ☐ Vaginal dryness/itching | No. |
| ☐ Sleeping problems (falling asleep, staying asleep, early waking, snoring) | No. |
| ☐ Urinary frequency | No. |
| ☐ Nipple discharge | Yes, just last week I noticed some milky discharge from my left breast. |
| ☐ Visual changes | No. |
| ☐ Headache | No. |
| ☐ Abdominal pain | No. |
| ☐ Sexual activity | Once a week on average with my husband. |
| ☐ Contraceptives | The same pills for eight years. |
| ☐ Pregnancies | I have one child; he is 10 years old. |
| ☐ Problems during pregnancy/delivery | No, it was a normal delivery, and my child is healthy. |
| ☐ Miscarriages/abortions | No. |
| ☐ Last Pap smear | Ten months ago. It was normal. |

| ☑ Question | Patient Response |
|---|---|
| ☐ History of abnormal Pap smears | No. |
| ☐ Current medications | None. |
| ☐ Past medical history | None. |
| ☐ Past surgical history | None. |
| ☐ Family history | My father and mother are healthy; my mother began menopause at age 55. |
| ☐ Occupation | Nurse. |
| ☐ Alcohol use | None. |
| ☐ Illicit drug use | Never. |
| ☐ Tobacco | No. |
| ☐ Exercise | I run two miles three times a week. |
| ☐ Drug allergies | No. |

## Physical Examination:

☐ Examinee washed his/her hands.
☐ Examinee asked permission to start the exam.
☐ Examinee used respectful draping.
☐ Examinee did not repeat painful maneuvers.

| ☑ Exam Component | Maneuver |
|---|---|
| ☐ Neck | Examined thyroid gland |
| ☐ CV exam | Auscultation |
| ☐ Pulmonary exam | Auscultation |
| ☐ Abdominal exam | Auscultation, percussion, palpation |
| ☐ Extremities | Inspection |
| ☐ Neurologic exam | Visual fields, extraocular movements, checked DTRs |

## Closure:

☐ Examinee discussed initial diagnostic impressions.
☐ Examinee discussed initial management plans:
    ☐ Diagnostic tests.
    ☐ Follow-up tests: Examinee mentioned the need for a pelvic and breast exam.
☐ Examinee asked if the patient has any other questions or concerns.

# PATIENT NOTE

**History**

**Physical Examination**

**Differential Diagnosis**

1.

2.

3.

4.

5.

**Diagnostic Workup**

1.

2.

3.

4.

5.

## History

**HPI:** 36 yo F c/o amenorrhea for 3 months. She recently noticed some milky discharge from her left breast as well as abnormal facial hair but denies visual changes or headache. She also describes oligomenorrhea, hypomenorrhea, and a 15-pound weight gain over the past year but denies dry skin, cold intolerance, voice change, constipation, depression, fatigue, or sleep problems. She also denies hot flushes and vaginal dryness or itching.

**OB/GYN:** Menarche at age 14. For the last year, menses have cycled every 5–6 weeks and lasted for 7 days, with decreased blood flow. Before that, menses cycled every 4 weeks. G1P1; 1 uncomplicated vaginal delivery 10 years ago. Last Pap smear 10 months ago; no history of abnormal Pap smears. Sexually active with husband once a week on average; uses OCPs for contraception.

**ROS:** Negative except as above.

**Allergies:** NKDA.

**Medicines:** None.

**PMH/PSH:** None.

**SH:** Denies tobacco, alcohol, or illicit drug use. Exercises regularly. Vegetarian; hasn't changed her diet recently.

**FH:** Mother had menopause at age 55.

## Physical Examination

Patient is in no acute distress.

**VS:** WNL.

**HEENT:** EOMI without diplopia or lid lag; visual fields full to confrontation.

**Neck:** No thyromegaly.

**Chest:** Clear breath sounds bilaterally.

**Heart:** RRR; normal S1/S2; no murmurs, rubs, or gallops.

**Abdomen:** Soft, nontender, nondistended, ⊕BS, no hepatosplenomegaly.

**Extremities:** No edema, no tremor.

**Neuro:** See HEENT. Normal DTRs in lower extremities bilaterally.

## Differential Diagnosis

1. Pregnancy
2. Hyperprolactinemia
3. Polycystic ovary syndrome (PCOS)
4. Thyroid disease
5. Premature ovarian failure
6. Asherman's syndrome

## Diagnostic Workup

1. Pelvic and breast exam
2. Urine hCG
3. LH/FSH
4. Prolactin, TSH
5. Electrolytes, glucose, BUN/Cr, ALT/bilirubin/ alkaline phosphatase
6. Testosterone, DHEAS
7. MRI—brain
8. Hysteroscopy

# CASE DISCUSSION

## Differential Diagnosis

- **Pregnancy:** This is the most common cause of secondary amenorrhea in women of childbearing age and should be ruled out during the initial evaluation.
- **Hyperprolactinemia:** This causes menstrual cycle disturbances, galactorrhea, and infertility. It may result from a variety of conditions, including pregnancy, hypothyroidism, renal failure, and cirrhosis, or it can be a side effect of medications. Roughly 70% of women with secondary amenorrhea and galactorrhea will have hyperprolactinemia.
- **PCOS:** This manifests variably as hirsutism, obesity, virilization, infertility, and glucose intolerance. Half of patients have amenorrhea (due to chronic anovulation). The patient's oligomenorrhea and hirsutism in the context of recent weight gain suggest this diagnosis.
- **Thyroid disease:** Hyper- and hypothyroidism can both cause menstrual irregularities, although amenorrhea is more commonly due to hypothyroidism. Except for galactorrhea and weight gain, the patient does not have other signs or symptoms of thyroid disease.
- **Premature ovarian failure:** This refers to primary hypogonadism that occurs before age 40. Causes include autoimmunity against the ovary, pelvic radiation therapy, chemotherapy, surgical bilateral oophorectomy, and familial factors. The patient's lack of menopausal symptoms (e.g., fatigue, insomnia, headache, diminished libido, depression, and hot flushes) makes this diagnosis unlikely.
- **Asherman's syndrome:** This describes amenorrhea due to endometrial scarring, which can occur following uterine infections. The vaginal estrogen effect is normal.

## Diagnostic Workup

- **Pelvic and breast exam:** Required to check for genital virilization (i.e., clitoromegaly), uterine or adnexal enlargement, and estrogen effect (via inspection of vaginal mucosa and Pap smear) and to elicit breast discharge.
- **Urine hCG:** To rule out pregnancy.
- **LH/FSH:** PCOS is a clinical diagnosis; an increased LH/FSH ratio is often seen but is neither necessary nor sufficient to make the diagnosis. Physiologically, increased levels of estrone (derived from obesity) are believed to suppress pituitary FSH, leading to a relative increase in LH. Constant LH stimulation of the ovary then results in anovulation (and often amenorrhea). An elevated FSH (> 40) is diagnostic for premature ovarian failure.
- **Prolactin, TSH:** To screen for hyperprolactinemia and thyroid disease. Free $T_4$ is also useful if hyperthyroidism (or central hypothyroidism) is suspected.
- **Electrolytes, glucose, BUN/Cr, ALT/bilirubin/alkaline phosphatase:** To check renal and hepatic function and to screen for evidence of hypercortisolism (e.g., high sodium and low potassium).
- **Testosterone, DHEAS:** To screen for hyperandrogenism when amenorrhea is accompanied by hirsutism and virilization. Mild elevations are often due to PCOS, but high levels may be due to ovarian or adrenal tumors.
- **MRI—brain:** Required to evaluate the pituitary region in patients suspected of having amenorrhea due to a hypothalamic or pituitary etiology (e.g., hyperprolactinemia).
- **Hysteroscopy:** To look for endometrial adhesions that are diagnostic for Asherman's syndrome.

## Opening Scenario

Stephanie McCall, a 28-year-old female, comes to the office complaining of pain during sex.

## Vital Signs

BP: 120/85 mmHg
Temp: 98.0°F (36.7°C)
RR: 13/minute
HR: 65/minute, regular

## Examinee Tasks

1. Take a focused history.
2. Perform a focused physical exam (do not perform rectal, genitourinary, or female breast exam).
3. Explain your clinical impression and workup plan to the patient.
4. Write the patient note after leaving the room.

## Checklist/SP Sheet

### PATIENT DESCRIPTION
Patient is a 28 yo F.

### NOTES FOR THE SP
None.

### CHALLENGING QUESTIONS TO ASK
When asked about vaginal discharge, ask, "Do you think I have a sexually transmitted disease?"

### SAMPLE EXAMINEE RESPONSE
"There are many causes of vaginal discharge, only some of which are due to sexually transmitted infections. I will try to look for clues by asking you more questions and examining you, and we will definitely send a sample of the discharge to the lab to check for infection."

## Examinee Checklist

### ENTRANCE:

☐ Examinee knocked on the door before entering.
☐ Examinee introduced self by name.
☐ Examinee identified his/her role or position.
☐ Examinee correctly used patient's name.
☐ Examinee made eye contact with the SP.

☐ Examinee showed compassion for your pain.

| ☑ Question | Patient Response |
|---|---|
| ☐ Chief complaint | I have been experiencing pain during sex. |
| ☐ Onset | Three months ago. |
| ☐ Describe pain | Aching and burning. |
| ☐ Timing | It happens every time I try to have sex. |
| ☐ Location | In the vaginal area. It starts on the outside, and I feel it on the inside with deep thrusting. |
| ☐ Vaginal discharge | Yes, recently. |
| ☐ Color/amount/smell | White, small amount every day (I don't have to wear a pad); it smells like fish. |
| ☐ Itching | Yes, a little bit. |
| ☐ Douching | No. |
| ☐ Last menstrual period | Two weeks ago. |
| ☐ Frequency of menstrual periods | Regular, every month; lasts for three days. |
| ☐ Pads/tampons changed a day | Three. |
| ☐ Painful periods | Yes, they have started to be painful over the past year. |
| ☐ Postcoital or intermenstrual bleeding | No. |
| ☐ Sexual partner | I have had the same boyfriend for the last year; before that I had a relationship with my ex-boyfriend for five years. |
| ☐ Contraception | I am using the patch. |
| ☐ Sexual desire | Good. |
| ☐ Conflicts with partner | No, we are pretty close. |
| ☐ Feeling safe at home | Yes, I have my own apartment. |
| ☐ History of physical, sexual, or emotional abuse | I don't usually talk about it, but I was raped in college, and that was when I contracted gonorrhea. |
| ☐ History of vaginal infections or STDs | I had gonorrhea 10 years ago in college. |
| ☐ Last Pap smear | Six months ago; it was normal. |
| ☐ History of abnormal Pap smears | No. |
| ☐ Depression/anxiety | No. |
| ☐ Hot flushes | No. |
| ☐ Vaginal dryness during intercourse | No. |
| ☐ Sleeping problems | No. |
| ☐ Urinary frequency/pain with urination | No. |

| ✓ **Question** | **Patient Response** |
|---|---|
| ☐ Pregnancies | I have never been pregnant. |
| ☐ Current medications | None. |
| ☐ Past medical history | None. |
| ☐ Past surgical history | None. |
| ☐ Family history | Both parents are healthy. |
| ☐ Occupation | Editor for a fashion magazine. |
| ☐ Alcohol use | A couple of beers on the weekends; sometimes a glass of wine on a romantic dinner. |
| ☐ CAGE questions | No (to all four). |
| ☐ Illicit drug use | Marijuana in college. |
| ☐ Tobacco | No. |
| ☐ Exercise | I swim and run regularly. |
| ☐ Drug allergies | No. |

## Physical Examination:

☐ Examinee washed his/her hands.

☐ Examinee asked permission to start the exam.

☐ Examinee used respectful draping.

☐ Examinee did not repeat painful maneuvers.

| ✓ **Exam Component** | **Maneuver** |
|---|---|
| ☐ CV exam | Auscultation |
| ☐ Pulmonary exam | Auscultation |
| ☐ Abdominal exam | Auscultation, percussion, palpation |

## Closure:

☐ Examinee discussed initial diagnostic impressions.

☐ Examinee discussed initial management plans:

   ☐ Diagnostic tests.

   ☐ Follow-up tests: Examinee mentioned the need for a pelvic exam.

☐ Examinee asked if the patient has any other questions or concerns.

# PATIENT NOTE

**History**

**Physical Examination**

| Differential Diagnosis | Diagnostic Workup |
| --- | --- |
| 1. | 1. |
| 2. | 2. |
| 3. | 3. |
| 4. | 4. |
| 5. | 5. |

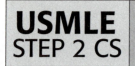

# PATIENT NOTE

## History

**HPI:** *28 yo F c/o pain during intercourse for 3 months, located both superficially and with deep thrusting. She also noticed a small, white vaginal discharge with a fishy odor, accompanied by mild vaginal pruritus. Denies postcoital or intermenstrual vaginal bleeding. She is sexually active with her boyfriend (only) for the past year, and her sexual desire is good. She feels safe at home and denies any conflicts with her partner. She also denies vaginal dryness, hot flushes, hirsutism, depression, fatigue, sleep problems, dysuria, and urinary frequency.*
**OB/GYN:** *G0P0. Last menstrual period 2 weeks ago; has regular menses but started to be painful over the past year. No history of abnormal Pap smears; most recent was 6 months ago. Uses patch for contraception.*
**ROS:** *Negative except as above.*
**Allergies:** *NKDA.*
**Medicines:** *None.*
**PMH:** *History of rape 10 years ago; subsequently contracted gonorrhea.*
**SH:** *No tobacco. Drinks a couple of beers on the weekends, occasional wine, CAGE 0/4, used marijuana in college. Exercises regularly.*
**FH:** *Noncontributory.*

## Physical Examination

*Patient is in no acute distress.*
**VS:** *WNL.*
**Chest:** *Clear breath sounds bilaterally.*
**Heart:** *RRR; normal S1/S2; no murmurs, rubs, or gallops.*
**Abdomen:** *Soft, nontender, nondistended, +BS, no hepatosplenomegaly.*

## Differential Diagnosis

1. Vulvovaginitis
2. Cervicitis
3. Endometriosis
4. Vulvodynia
5. Domestic violence
6. Pelvic tumor
7. Vaginismus

## Diagnostic Workup

1. Pelvic exam
2. Wet mount, KOH prep, "whiff" test
3. Cervical cultures (chlamydia and gonorrhea DNA probes)
4. U/S—pelvis
5. MRI—pelvis
6. Laparoscopy

## CASE DISCUSSION

### Differential Diagnosis

- **Vulvovaginitis:** This describes infection or inflammation of the vagina. Etiologies include pathogens, allergic or contact reactions, or friction from intercourse. The presence of vaginal discharge (accompanied by a fishy odor and pruritus) makes this a likely diagnosis.
- **Cervicitis:** The presence of vaginal discharge and pain with deep thrusting suggests infection or inflammation of the cervix.
- **Endometriosis:** This describes abnormal ectopic endometrial tissue, which can cause inflammation and scarring in the lower pelvis. Endometriosis may account for the patient's dysmenorrhea over the past year and, if so, could also cause dyspareunia with deep thrusting. Her history of gonorrhea infection (if it caused PID) also puts her at risk for pelvic scarring and subsequent dyspareunia (due to impaired mobility of pelvic organs).
- **Vulvodynia:** This is the leading cause of dyspareunia in premenopausal women but is not well understood. Pain may be constant or intermittent, focal or diffuse, and superficial or deep. Physical findings are often absent, making it a diagnosis of exclusion. However, vulvar erythema can be seen in a subset of vulvodynia termed *vulvar vestibulitis.*
- **Domestic violence:** Physicians must screen for this in any woman presenting with dyspareunia. Serial screening is required, as victims may not disclose this history initially.
- **Pelvic tumor:** This could account for the patient's pain with deep thrusting and possibly for her history of dysmenorrhea. However, pelvic tumors are not associated with vaginal discharge and pruritus.
- **Vaginismus:** This describes severe involuntary spasm of muscles around the introitus and often results from fear, pain, or sexual or psychological trauma. The muscle contractions generally preclude penetration. Although this patient was raped in the past, she does not describe the muscle contractions characteristic of vaginismus.

### Diagnostic Workup

- **Pelvic exam:** To localize and reproduce the pain or discomfort and to determine if any pathology is present. A complete exam includes external genital inspection and palpation, speculum exam, and bimanual and rectal exam.
- **Wet mount, KOH prep, "whiff" test:** The vaginal discharge is examined microscopically. The presence of epithelial cells covered with bacteria (clue cells) suggests bacterial vaginosis, and the presence of hyphae and spores indicates candidal infection. Motile organisms are seen in trichomonal infection. A "fishy" odor after exposure of the discharge to a drop of potassium hydroxide is characteristic of bacterial vaginosis.
- **Cervical cultures:** To diagnose chlamydia, gonorrhea, and occasionally HSV infection (the latter is characterized by the presence of vesicles or ulcers on the cervix).
- **Imaging studies:** U/S and MRI are useful to assess the size and positioning of pelvic organs and to help rule out masses or other pathology.
- **Laparoscopy:** This is the gold standard test used to confirm a clinical diagnosis of endometriosis.

## Opening Scenario

Rick Meyer, a 51-year-old male construction worker, comes to the office complaining of back pain.

## Vital Signs

**BP:** 120/85 mmHg
**Temp:** 98.2°F (36.8°C)
**RR:** 20/minute
**HR:** 80/minute, regular

## Examinee Tasks

1. Take a focused history.
2. Perform a focused physical exam (do not perform rectal, genitourinary, or female breast exam).
3. Explain your clinical impression and workup plan to the patient.
4. Write the patient note after leaving the room.

## Checklist/SP Sheet

### PATIENT DESCRIPTION

Patient is a 51 yo M who lives with his girlfriend.

### NOTES FOR THE SP

- Pretend that you have paraspinal lower back tenderness when examined.
- Show normal reflexes, sensation, and strength in both lower extremities.
- Lean forward slightly when walking.

### CHALLENGING QUESTIONS TO ASK

"I don't think I can go to work, doctor. Can you write a letter to my boss so that I can have some days off?"

### SAMPLE EXAMINEE RESPONSE

"You're right, heavy construction work can worsen your back pain or cause it to heal more slowly. I will ask your boss to reassign you to light duty for a while."

## Examinee Checklist

### ENTRANCE:

- ☐ Examinee knocked on the door before entering.
- ☐ Examinee introduced self by name.
- ☐ Examinee identified his/her role or position.
- ☐ Examinee correctly used patient's name.
- ☐ Examinee made eye contact with the SP.

☐  Examinee showed compassion for your pain.

| ☑ Question | Patient Response |
| --- | --- |
| ☐ Chief complaint | Pain in my back. |
| ☐ Onset | One week ago. |
| ☐ Associated/precipitating events | I was lifting some heavy boxes; then my back started hurting right away. |
| ☐ Progression | It has been the same. |
| ☐ Severity on a scale | 8/10. |
| ☐ Location | The middle of my lower back. |
| ☐ Radiation | To my left thigh and sometimes reaches my left foot. |
| ☐ Quality | Sharp. |
| ☐ Alleviating factors | Lying still in bed. |
| ☐ Exacerbating factors | Walking, sitting for a long time, coughing. |
| ☐ Weakness/numbness | None. |
| ☐ Difficulty urinating | I noticed that over the last six months I have had to strain to be able to urinate. Sometimes I feel that I didn't empty my bladder fully. |
| ☐ Urinary or fecal incontinence | No. |
| ☐ Fever, night sweats, weight loss | No. |
| ☐ History of back pain in the past | Well, for the past year I have been having back pain on and off, mainly when I walk. It is usually accompanied by pain in my legs. That pain goes away when I stop walking and sit down. |
| ☐ Current medications | I take ibuprofen. It helps, but the pain is still there. |
| ☐ Past medical history | None. |
| ☐ Past surgical history | None. |
| ☐ Family history | My father died of a heart attack at age 65, and my mother is healthy. |
| ☐ Occupation | Construction worker. |
| ☐ Alcohol use | Yes, a couple of beers on the weekends. |
| ☐ CAGE questions | No (to all four). |
| ☐ Illicit drug use | Never. |
| ☐ Tobacco | Yes, one pack a day for the last 18 years. |
| ☐ Drug allergies | Penicillin, causes rash. |

## Physical Examination:

☐ Examinee washed his/her hands.

☐ Examinee asked permission to start the exam.

☐ Examinee used respectful draping.

☐ Examinee did not repeat painful maneuvers.

| ☑ Exam Component | Maneuver |
| --- | --- |
| ☐ Back | Inspection, palpation, range of motion |
| ☐ Extremities | Inspection, palpation of peripheral pulses, hip exam |
| ☐ Neurologic exam | Motor, DTRs, Babinski's sign, gait (including toe and heel walking), passive straight leg raising, sensory |

## Closure:

☐ Examinee discussed initial diagnostic impressions.

☐ Examinee discussed initial management plans:

    ☐ Diagnostic tests.

    ☐ Follow-up tests: Examinee mentioned the need for a rectal exam.

☐ Examinee asked if the patient has any other questions or concerns.

# PATIENT NOTE

**History**

**Physical Examination**

**Differential Diagnosis**

1.

2.

3.

4.

5.

**Diagnostic Workup**

1.

2.

3.

4.

5.

## History

**HPI:** *The patient is a 51 yo construction worker complaining of lower back pain that started after lifting heavy boxes 1 week ago. The pain is 8/10, is sharp, and radiates to the left thigh and sometimes to the left foot. Pain worsens with movement, cough, and sitting for a long time. Pain is relieved by lying still and partially by ibuprofen. He denies urinary or stool incontinence or weakness or loss of sensation in the lower extremities. No fever, night sweats, or weight loss. He does report difficulty urinating and incomplete emptying of the bladder for 6 months as well as a 1-year history of intermittent lower back pain and leg pain with ambulation that resolves with sitting.*

**ROS:** *Negative except as above.*

**Allergies:** *Penicillin (causes rash).*

**PMH:** *None.*

**PSH:** *None.*

**SH:** *One PPD for 18 years, drinks a couple of beers on weekends, CAGE 0/4.*

**FH:** *Noncontributory.*

## Physical Examination

*Patient is in mild distress due to back pain.*

**Back:** *Mild paraspinal muscle tenderness bilaterally, normal range of motion. No warmth or erythema.*

**Extremities:** *2+ popliteal, dorsalis pedis, and posterior tibial pulses bilaterally. Hips normal, nontender range of motion bilaterally.*

**Neuro:** *Motor: Strength 5/5 throughout, including left great toe dorsiflexion. DTRs: 2+ symmetric, ⊖Babinski bilaterally. Gait: Normal (including toe and heel walking), although walks with back slightly bent forward. Straight leg raising negative bilaterally. Sensation: Intact.*

## Differential Diagnosis

1. Disk herniation
2. Lumbar muscle strain
3. Degenerative arthritis
4. Lumbar spinal stenosis
5. Metastatic prostate cancer
6. Multiple myeloma
7. Malingering

## Diagnostic Workup

1. Rectal exam
2. XR—L-spine
3. MRI—L-spine
4. PSA
5. CBC, calcium, BUN/Cr
6. SPEP/UPEP

# CASE DISCUSSION

## Differential Diagnosis

- **Disk herniation:** Low back pain radiating down the buttock and below the knee suggests nerve root irritation due to disk herniation. However, this pattern is nonspecific and can also be caused by sacroiliitis, facet joint degenerative arthritis, spinal stenosis, or other causes of sciatica. Most disk herniations occur at the L4–L5 or L5–S1 vertebral levels. These nerve roots are quickly assessed by checking the knee-jerk reflex (L4), great toe dorsiflexion (L5), and ankle-jerk reflex (S1). Ipsilateral straight leg raising that produces radicular symptoms (with the leg raised < 60 degrees) is highly sensitive but is nonspecific in herniations at these levels. This patient may have disk herniation but has no objective evidence of neurologic compromise at this point.
- **Lumbar muscle strain:** This often follows strenuous or unusual exertion, but pain usually does not radiate to the extremities. Paraspinal muscle tenderness is often present.
- **Degenerative arthritis:** Degenerative back diseases are common, and classically pain is exacerbated by activity and alleviated by rest. Radicular symptoms may be present.
- **Lumbar spinal stenosis:** This is most often seen in patients > 60 years of age. They present with gradual onset of back pain that radiates to the buttocks and legs with or without leg numbness and weakness. Pain usually occurs with walking or prolonged standing and subsides by sitting or leaning forward (as in this case).
- **Metastatic prostate cancer:** The most common cancers leading to vertebral body metastasis are prostate, breast, lung, multiple myeloma, and lymphoma. In metastatic disease, patients complain of gradual-onset (or occasionally acute in the case of pathologic fracture) back pain with or without neurologic symptoms. Pain may be worse at night and unrelieved by rest. This patient's urinary symptoms may be a sign of prostatic disease.
- **Multiple myeloma:** Typically, patients are > 50 years of age. Back and bone pain may be the only presenting complaint. Anemia, neuropathy, hypercalcemia, and renal failure are also common.
- **Malingering:** This is defined as intentional faking of symptoms for secondary gain (e.g., getting out of work).

## Diagnostic Workup

The history and physical exam are often all that is required, as the majority of patients with low back pain will improve within four weeks. Patients who require more extensive or urgent evaluation are those suspected of having pain caused by infection, cancer, abdominal aortic aneurysm, or neurologic emergency (e.g., cauda equina syndrome).

- **Rectal exam (including "saddle area" sensory exam):** To evaluate the prostate, rectal sphincter tone, and integrity of sacral nerve roots.
- **XR–L-spine:** Can show evidence of vertebral osteomyelitis, cancer, or fractures. Degenerative changes are expected in older patients and correlate poorly with clinical symptoms.
- **MRI–L-spine:** Provides the best anatomical detail and is the test of choice for suspected herniation, infection, or malignancy. Remember that asymptomatic disk herniation is common, so its presence does not necessarily correlate with clinical disease.
- **PSA:** Screening test for prostate cancer.
- **CBC, calcium, BUN/Cr:** To detect anemia, hypercalcemia, and renal failure, which may be clues to underlying multiple myeloma.
- **SPEP/UPEP:** To detect a monoclonal paraprotein in myeloma.

# Acronyms and Abbreviations

| Abbreviation | Meaning |
|---|---|
| ABG | arterial blood gas |
| ACE | angiotensin-converting enzyme |
| ACh | acetylcholine |
| ADLs | activities of daily living |
| AFB | acid-fast bacillus |
| AIDS | acquired immunodeficiency syndrome |
| ALT | alanine aminotransferase |
| ANA | antinuclear antibody |
| AP | anteroposterior |
| AST | aspartate aminotransferase |
| AXR | abdominal x-ray |
| BP | blood pressure |
| BPH | benign prostatic hypertrophy |
| BPPV | benign paroxysmal positional vertigo |
| BS | bowel sounds |
| BUN | blood urea nitrogen |
| c/o | complains of |
| CA 19-9 | carbohydrate antigen 19-9 |
| CABG | coronary artery bypass graft |
| C-ANCA | cytoplasmic antineutrophil cytoplasmic antibody |
| CBC | complete blood count |
| CD | cluster of differentiation |
| CEA | carcinoembryonic antigen |
| CHF | congestive heart failure |
| CMV | cytomegalovirus |
| CN | cranial nerve |
| CNS | central nervous system |
| COM | communication [CSE score] |
| COPD | chronic obstructive pulmonary disease |
| CPK | creatine phosphokinase |
| CPK-MB | creatine phosphokinase, MB fraction |
| Cr | creatinine |
| CREST | calcinosis, Raynaud's phenomenon, esophageal dysmotility, sclerodactyly, telangiectasia [syndrome] |
| CRP | C-reactive protein |
| CSA | Clinical Skills Assessment |
| CS | Clinical Skills |
| CSF | cerebrospinal fluid |
| CT | computed tomography |
| CV | cardiovascular |

| Abbreviation | Meaning |
|---|---|
| CVA | costovertebral angle or cerebrovascular accident |
| CXR | chest x-ray |
| D&C | dilatation and curettage |
| DDAVP | 1-deamino (8-D-arginine) vasopressin |
| DEXA | dual-energy x-ray absorptiometry |
| DFA | direct fluorescent antibody [test] |
| DG | data gathering [CSE score] |
| DHEAS | dehydroepiandrosterone sulfate |
| DI | diabetes insipidus |
| DIC | disseminated intravascular coagulation |
| DM | diabetes mellitus |
| DNA | deoxyribonucleic acid |
| dsDNA | double-stranded deoxyribonucleic acid |
| DTR | deep tendon reflex |
| DVT | deep venous thrombosis |
| EBNA | Epstein-Barr nuclear antigen |
| EBV | Epstein-Barr virus |
| ECFMG | Educational Commission for Foreign Medical Graduates |
| ECG | electrocardiogram |
| ED | erectile dysfunction |
| EEG | electroencephalogram |
| EMG | electromyogram |
| ENT | ear, nose, and throat |
| EOMI | extraocular movements intact |
| ER | emergency room |
| ERCP | endoscopic retrograde cholangiopancreatography |
| ESR | erythrocyte sedimentation rate |
| ET | essential tremor |
| EtOH | ethyl alcohol |
| FH | family history |
| FSH | follicle-stimulating hormone |
| FSMB | Federation of State Medical Boards |
| $FT_4$ | free thyroxine |
| GERD | gastroesophageal reflux disease |
| GI | gastrointestinal |
| hCG | human chorionic gonadotropin |
| HCTZ | hydrochlorothiazide |
| HEENT | head, eyes, ears, nose, and throat |
| HgA1c | hemoglobin A1c |

| Abbreviation | Meaning |
|---|---|
| HIDA | hepatobiliary iminodiacetic acid [scan] |
| HIV | human immunodeficiency virus |
| HPI | history of present illness |
| HR | heart rate |
| HRT | hormone replacement therapy |
| HSV | herpes simplex virus |
| IADLs | instrumental activities of daily living |
| ICE | integrated clinical encounter [CSE score] |
| Ig | immunoglobulin |
| IMED | International Medical Education Directory |
| IMG | international medical graduate |
| IPS | interpersonal skills [CSE score] |
| IV | intravenous |
| IVDU | intravenous drug use |
| IVP | intravenous pyelography |
| IWA | interactive Web application |
| JVD | jugular venous distention |
| KOH | potassium hydroxide |
| LDH | lactose dehydrogenase |
| LH | luteinizing hormone |
| LLQ | left lower quadrant |
| LOC | loss of consciousness |
| LP | lumbar puncture |
| LUQ | left upper quadrant |
| LVH | left ventricular hypertrophy |
| MCP | metacarpophalangeal [joint] |
| MDI | metered-dose inhaler |
| MI | myocardial infarction |
| MRA | magnetic resonance angiography |
| MRCP | magnetic resonance cholangiopancreatography |
| MRI | magnetic resonance imaging |
| MS | multiple sclerosis |
| MTP | metatarsophalangeal [joint] |
| NBME | National Board of Medical Examiners |
| NC/AT | normocephalic/atraumatic |
| NKDA | no known drug allergies |
| NRMP | National Residency Matching Program |
| NSAID | nonsteroidal anti-inflammatory drug |
| OCP | oral contraceptive pill |
| OTC | over the counter |
| PCOS | polycystic ovary syndrome |
| PCP | *Pneumocystic carinii* pneumonia |
| PCR | polymerase chain reaction |
| PD | Parkinson's disease |
| PERRLA | pupils equal, round, and reactive to light and accommodation |
| PFT | pulmonary function test |
| PID | pelvic inflammatory disease |
| PMH | past medical history |

| Abbreviation | Meaning |
|---|---|
| PMI | point of maximal impulse |
| PN | patient note |
| PPD | pack per day, purified protein derivative [tuberculin skin test] |
| prn | pro re nata [as needed] |
| PSA | prostate-specific antigen |
| PSH | past surgical history |
| PT | prothrombin time |
| PTSD | post-traumatic stress disorder |
| PTT | partial thromboplastin time |
| PUD | peptic ulcer disease |
| RF | rheumatoid factor |
| RLQ | right lower quadrant |
| ROS | review of systems |
| RPR | rapid plasma reagin |
| RR | respiratory rate |
| RRR | regular rate and rhythm |
| RUQ | right upper quadrant |
| SH | social history |
| SIADH | syndrome of inappropriate antidiuretic hormone |
| SLE | systemic lupus erythematosus |
| SP | standardized patient |
| SPECT | single-photon emission computed tomography |
| SPEP | serum protein electrophoresis |
| SSRI | selective serotonin reuptake inhibitor |
| STD | sexually transmitted disease |
| TB | tuberculosis |
| TEE | transesophageal echocardiography |
| TIA | transient ischemic attack |
| TIBC | total iron-binding capacity |
| TM | tympanic membrane |
| TMJ | temporomandibular joint |
| TOEFL | Test of English as a Foreign Language |
| TSE | test of spoken English |
| TSH | thyroid-stimulating hormone |
| TTE | transthoracic echocardiography |
| UA | urinalysis |
| UPEP | urine protein electrophoresis |
| URI | upper respiratory infection |
| U/S | ultrasound |
| UTD | up to date [vaccinations] |
| UTI | urinary tract infection |
| VA | Veterans Administration |
| VCA | virus capsid antigen |
| VDRL | Venereal Disease Research Laboratory |
| V/Q | ventilation-perfusion [scan] |
| VS | vital signs |
| WBC | white blood cell |
| WNL | within normal limits |
| XR | x-ray |
| yo | year old |

# Index

271

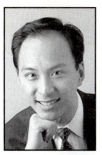
Tao Le, MD

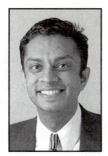
Vikas Bhushan, MD

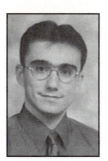
Fadi Abu Shahin, MD

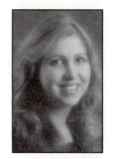
Mae Sheikh-Ali, MD

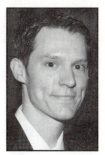
L. David Martin, MD

**Tao Le, MD**

Dr. Le has led multiple medical education projects over the past thirteen years. As a medical student, he was editor-in-chief of the University of California, San Francisco *Synapse,* a university newspaper with a weekly circulation of 9000. Subsequently, he authored *First Aid for the Wards* and *First Aid for the Match* and led the most recent revision of *First Aid for the USMLE Step 2.* At Yale, he was a regular guest lecturer on the USMLE review courses and an adviser to the Yale University School of Medicine curriculum committee. Dr. Le earned his medical degree from the University of California, San Francisco in 1996 and completed his residency training and board certification in internal medicine at Yale–New Haven Hospital. Dr. Le subsequently went on to cofound Medsn and served as its Chief Medical Officer. He is currently pursuing research in asthma education as a fellow in allergy and clinical immunology at the Johns Hopkins Asthma and Allergy Center.

**Vikas Bhushan, MD**

Dr. Bhushan is a world-renowned author, publisher, entrepreneur, and board-certified diagnostic radiologist who resides in Los Angeles, California. Dr. Bhushan conceived and authored the original *First Aid for the USMLE Step 1* in 1992, which, after 11 consecutive editions, has become the most popular medical review book in the world. Following this, he coauthored three additional *First Aid* books as well as developed the highly acclaimed 17-title *Underground Clinical Vignettes* series. He completed his training in diagnostic radiology at the University of California, Los Angeles. Dr. Bhushan has more than 13 years of entrepreneurial experience and started two successful software and publishing companies prior to cofounding Medsn. He has worked directly with dozens of medical school faculty, colleagues, and consultants and corresponded with thousands of medical students from around the world. Dr. Bhushan earned his bachelor's degree in biochemistry from the University of California, Berkeley, and his MD with thesis from the University of California, San Francisco.

**Fadi Abu Shahin, MD**

Dr. Abu Shahin is currently a resident of Obstetrics and Gynecology at Northwestern University in Chicago. If not delivering babies in Prentice Women's Hospital, he spends his time playing classic guitar or watching movies. He is a distinguished graduate of Damascus University Medical School in Syria. He was a postdoctoral fellow in the Department of Obstetrics and Gynecology at Yale University. His research was focused on ovarian cancer and the effects of estrogen on the immune system. He has been a contributor, editor, and author of several editions of the *First Aid for the USMLE* and the *Underground Clinical Vignettes* series. Fadi speaks Arabic, English, French, and Spanish. He has also started tackling the Japanese language. His goal is to become a gynecologic oncologist in an academic institution.

**Mae Sheikh-Ali, MD**

Dr. Sheikh-Ali is currently a resident in internal medicine at Drexel University College of Medicine in Philadelphia. After graduating from Damascus University School of Medicine in Syria, she worked as a physician at the International School in Damascus, where she provided medical care to the students. The following year, she worked with the Emergency and Medical Service Agency as an on-call emergency physician. There she became proficient at approaching difficult problems and handling them expeditiously. She is an editor and contributing author of several editions of the *First Aid for the USMLE* and the *Underground Clinical Vignettes* series. Dr. Sheikh-Ali enjoys taking an active role in medical education by teaching and empowering medical students, residents, as well as patients. Her goal is to pursue an academic career in Endocrinology with a focus on diabetes prevention and management. She will be starting her fellowship in Endocrinology at the Mayo Clinic, Florida in 2005.

**L. David Martin, MD**

Dr. Martin is an instructor at the Johns Hopkins University School of Medicine. He completed his undergraduate and medical education at Duke University and Wake Forest/Bowman Gray School of Medicine, and recently completed primary care internal medicine residency training at Johns Hopkins Bayview Medical Center. His interests include HIV and addiction medicine, medical education and teaching, and revolutionizing the doctor's black bag with modern tools of the trade. He will serve as a chief resident at Bayview during 2004–2005.

# ABOUT THE AUTHORS

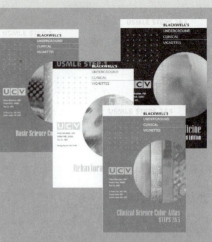